Men's Fitness
COMPLETE GUIDE TO
ABS

Contributors Pete Muir, Jon Lipsey, Lucy Miller, Joe Warner
Design Ian Jackson
Sub Editors Emma Hartfield, Chris Miller
Photography Tom Miles, Michael E
Model Toby Rowland@Nevs

With thanks to

FitnessFirst

fitnessfirst.co.uk

For more information on Men's Fitness magazine, go to **mensfitnessmagazine.co.uk**
To subscribe call **0844 844 0081**

Copyright Dennis Publishing Ltd. Licensed by Felden 2008

Sports Nutrition

What every gym user should know

Using the right sports nutrition products can help you build muscle, gain strength, lose fat and get into shape more easily. There are so many products out there and it can often seem confusing. This guide is designed to help you to choose the right products for your goal.

Fat Management

Stripping away fat and exposing your six-pack can be made so much easier by adding **Pyro-MX Leanburn**® to your training and eating plan. Recent fat management research found that ingredients like citrus aurantium, guarana, green tea, cayenne and l-carnitine increase fat oxidation and help you to burn fat when used in conjunction with exercise. **Pyro-MX Leanburn**® contains optimum amounts of these ingredients, as well as an effective carb-blocker, tyrosine and vitamin B5. If your goal is to get lean and ripped, **Pyro-MX Leanburn**® is for you!

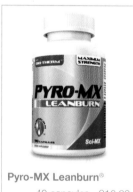

Pyro-MX Leanburn®

40 capsules - £16.99
90 capsules - £27.99
180 capsules - £42.99

- Use in conjunction with your exercise and eating plan to accelerate fat loss.
- All active ingredients are from completely natural sources.

Special Online Offer

Buy any 3 items and save 20%

Visit www.sci-mx.co.uk today

Protein Powder

When training with weights, your body requires high levels of protein to maintain and grow lean muscle. It takes just a few hours for your body to use up the protein supplied in your diet and, once metabolised, your muscles start to use amino acids that are in muscle tissue. This is known as muscle wastage or catabolism. Sci-MX's gradual release **GRS-5 Protein System**™ is specifically designed to ensure that muscles are supplied with protein over a sustained period (both day and night), preventing muscle wastage and boosting muscle growth.

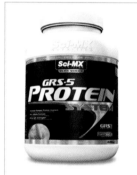

GRS-5 Protein System™
Available in Banana, Chocolate, Choc-Mint, Strawberry and Vanilla.

1kg (24 serv.) - £27.99
2.28kg (40 serv.) - £54.99

- **40g GRS-5**™ **Gradual Release Protein*** - consists of a blend of rapidly absorbed whey proteins and gradually released milk, egg and soy protein.
- **100mg of Aminogen**®* - a revolutionary new US developed and researched compound that has proven to boost protein absorption and retention.
- **OptiZyme**™ **Digestive Enzyme Package** - helps even the most sensitive stomach to digest protein so that none is wasted or passes through the system.

Muscle and Size

Omni-MX™ is a new generation 'all-in-one' lean muscle building formulation that combines the most effective ingredients for building lean, defined muscle. With all the different muscle building ingredients available it can be difficult understanding what each one does, how effective it is, and how it works. **Omni-MX**™ eliminates the confusion by supplying a perfectly synergised blend of ingredients that are tried and tested! **Omni-MX**™ will help you to pack on rock solid muscle when combined with weight training, with results showing in as little as 7 days!

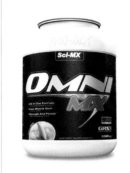

Omni-MX™
Available in Banana, Chocolate and Strawberry.
1.68kg (24 serv.) - £47.99

- **70g GRS-5**™ **Gradual Release Protein**[†] - muscles crave protein from any form of training and without enough protein in your diet your muscles simply wont grow! 70 grams of GRS-5™ protein per day ensures that your body has enough protein to grow.

- **10g Creatine**[†] - increases strength, size and explosiveness when combined with weight training. Sci-MX uses the purest form of creatine available, so no cramps or indigestion.

- **2g Beta-Alanine**[†] - helps build muscle quicker and works in synergy with creatine when weight training.

- **10g L-Glutamine**[†] - training depletes muscle glutamine levels rapidly, which causes muscle breakdown. 10 grams a day helps to prevent this.

- **3g HMB**[†] - the quicker you recover from training, the more muscle you will gain. HMB is a well researched and highly respected recovery agent.

- **23g Omni-Mino**™ **Growth Complex**[†] - unique to Sci-MX, Omni-Mino™ contains a combination of BCAAs, natural T boosting ecdysterone, chromium and Bioperine™ which together boost muscle building.

Lean Muscle Building Meal Replacement

One of the best ways to help lose fat, build muscle and boost your metabolism is to eat six modest meals per day - this is how we evolved to eat. Eating frequently activates primal survival mechanisms that tell our bodies that we do not need to store fat or slow down. Preparing six meals a day is impractical, which is why a meal replacement formula can be used to replace two or three solid food meals. **Lean Grow MRF**™ is ideal for active gym users who do not have the time to prepare six meals a day.

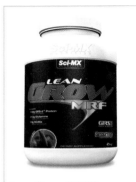

Lean Grow MRF™
Available in Chocolate, Strawberry and Vanilla.
1kg (9 serv.) - £21.99
2kg (18 serv.) - £36.99
5kg (45 serv.) - £69.99

- Provides the equivalent of 1½ chicken breasts, a small bowl of brown rice and all the vitamins and minerals which typically exist in a variety of vegetables and fruit*.

- Why not buy a few extra shaker bottles, add a serving to an empty shaker and take it with you to work? Just add water, shake and drink at meal times. Nice and easy!

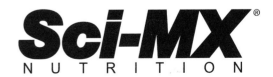

Let us help you avoid confusion and choose the right product for your goal

www.sci-mx.co.uk

FREE next working day delivery on orders over £30[‡]

Sci-MX®
N U T R I T I O N

Contents

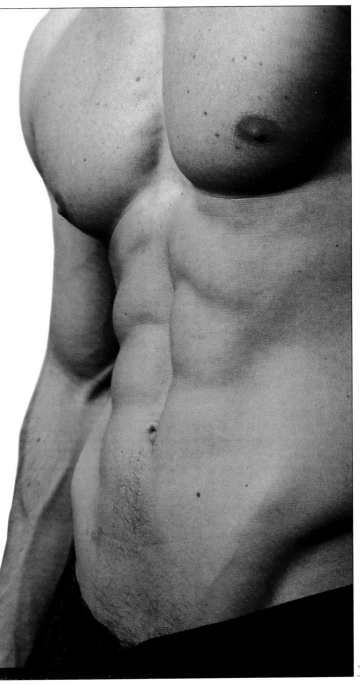

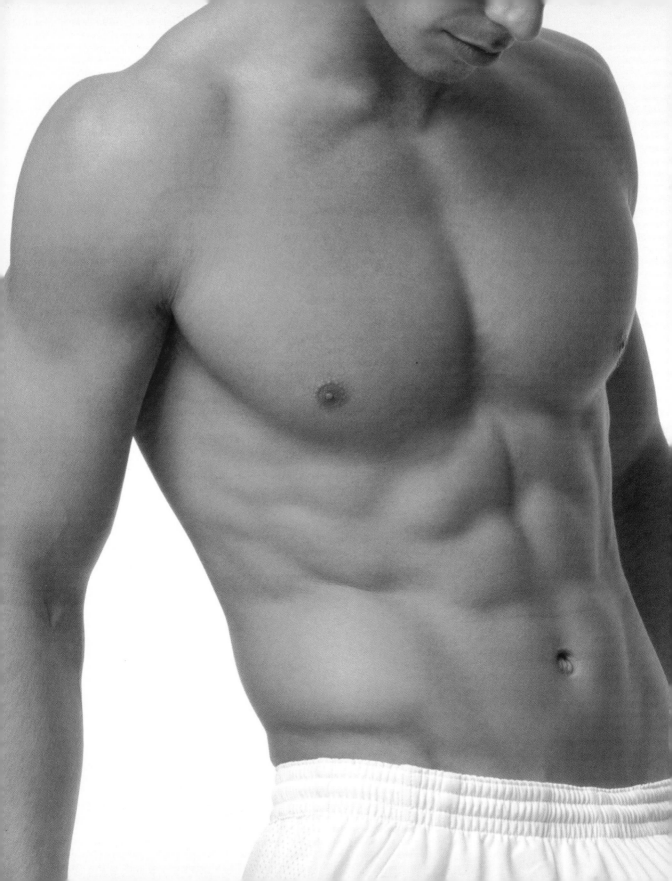

Your six-pack starts here

Read on for essential information on building a muscular stomach

Welcome to the *Complete Guide To Abs*, the ultimate training resource for anyone who wants to sculpt a six-pack. For many men, having a chiselled mid-section is their number one fitness goal. That's partly because rippling abs are popular with the ladies but also because they give you huge practical benefits.

Your core – the muscles around your midsection – is the link between your upper and lower body. So a strong core, including strong abs, is vital for all heavy lifting movements and in most dynamic sports. Building a six-pack can also help maintain good posture and prevent back pain.

An important part of developing your abs is to make sure that you get rid of excess flab around your stomach, which is where men are most likely to store fat. After all, you can have strong muscles but if they're buried under a layer of lard, you're not going to see the

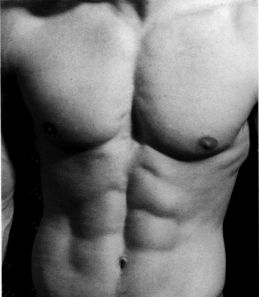

hard-earned results of your efforts. This guide will show you how to strip away fat while simultaneously building muscle – a simple concept but you need to do it right.

What's in this guide?

The biggest mistake people make when training their abs is thinking that doing endless crunches will give them a six-pack. It won't. Instead, you need to work your abs in different ways as part of a progressive training plan so that you continue to stimulate your muscles into new growth. To guide you through that process we look at the basic science behind building a six-pack as well as giving you our top abs tips and exploding common myths.

Performing a wide variety of exercises is key to developing muscle and the '72 Abs Moves' section (from p26) will give you the exercise arsenal you need to keep your training fresh. The three-part workout guide involves all the major muscle groups, with an emphasis on abs, to strip away fat and maximise your training effect. Finally, we've included a nutrition section with tips on eating for a six-pack, a guide to supplements and meal plans to complement your training and avoid piling that flab back on.

Start now and you'll soon have the stomach you've always wanted.

TURN OVER FOR MORE ABS-BUILDING TIPS

The science of abs

There's more to getting great abs than simply banging out crunches. Here's everything you need to know to reveal your six-pack

Here at *MF* the question we are asked most frequently is 'How can I get a six-pack?' The abdominals are the Top Trump trophy muscles and the ones that drive women wild – but that doesn't mean they're just for show. Our obsession with abs is justified because they are essential for making us fitter, stronger and faster. The abs may have come to symbolise masculinity but they also hold the key to beating your personal bests, whether you're in the park or the gym.

Six-pack science

If you want to build an impressive six-pack, you'll need to crank out a thousand crunches a week, right? Actually, no. We all have a six-pack underneath our body fat because our abs are crisscrossed by connective tissue that makes them look as if they're made up of separate segments. In order to make your six-pack more defined you have to increase the size of these muscle 'segments'. To do this, the basic principles of weight training apply.

You need to exhaust your abs by lifting a heavy load in a short, intense workout. You should then allow at least 48 hours for them to recover and grow before their next workout. You should also eat 1.5g–2g of lean protein per kilogram of your bodyweight as part of your normal diet when building muscle. Once you've built some muscular endurance in your abs with normal crunches, you need to add some extra resistance by holding a medicine ball, weight plate or dumb-bell across your chest.

This approach will develop the muscle underneath your layer of belly fat, but the fat itself will remain. Crunches or sit-ups alone will never burn off your beer belly. In fact, scientists with far too much time on their hands at the University of Virginia worked out that it would take 250,000 crunches to burn one pound of lard, by which time you would probably have died of boredom anyway.

In any case, this pound of fat would come off your entire body, not just the area around your abs. You can't burn fat from around your middle simply by working a specific area of your body, and it takes a significant overall reduction in your body fat percentage to uncover your abs. The best way to achieve this is still the old-fashioned way, with cardiovascular exercise.

Before you sign up for a marathon bear in mind that short, intense cardio workouts are better at torching calories and are less likely to burn off muscle. In fact, three 30-minute sessions per week of short-burst, intense cardio (combined with a diet low in saturated fat and processed carbs) can control body fat. Try

> **You will give your abs a fresh challenge and improve condition by hitting them from different angles**

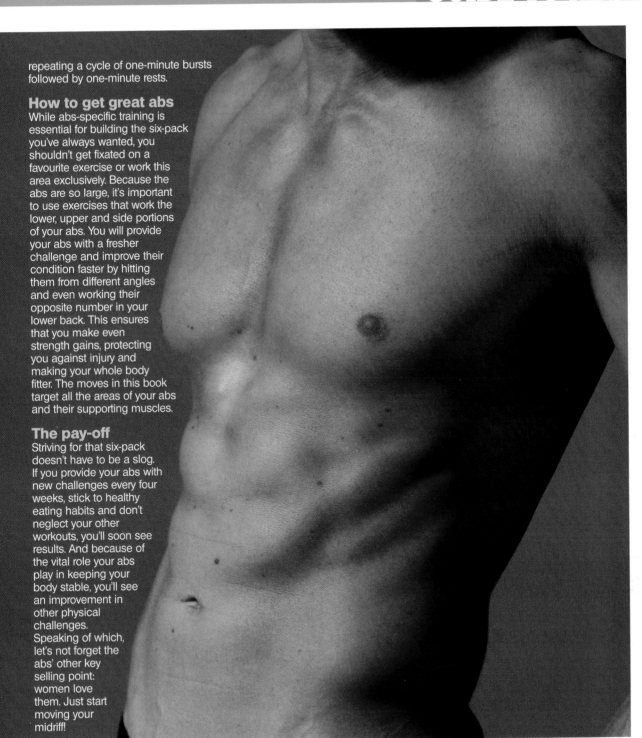

repeating a cycle of one-minute bursts followed by one-minute rests.

How to get great abs

While abs-specific training is essential for building the six-pack you've always wanted, you shouldn't get fixated on a favourite exercise or work this area exclusively. Because the abs are so large, it's important to use exercises that work the lower, upper and side portions of your abs. You will provide your abs with a fresher challenge and improve their condition faster by hitting them from different angles and even working their opposite number in your lower back. This ensures that you make even strength gains, protecting you against injury and making your whole body fitter. The moves in this book target all the areas of your abs and their supporting muscles.

The pay-off

Striving for that six-pack doesn't have to be a slog. If you provide your abs with new challenges every four weeks, stick to healthy eating habits and don't neglect your other workouts, you'll soon see results. And because of the vital role your abs play in keeping your body stable, you'll see an improvement in other physical challenges. Speaking of which, let's not forget the abs' other key selling point: women love them. Just start moving your midriff!

Abs anatomy

There's a lot more to that area under your shirt than just skin and flab

The term 'abs' causes some confusion. Although they are almost always referred to in the plural, and they look like a group of muscles, the abs consist of a single sheet that connects the top of your pelvic bone to the bottom of your ribcage. Hard connective tissue marks out eight 'segments', forming a visible six-pack (or eight-pack, if you're lucky).

But the abs are only part of the story – they're the standard bearer for the group of muscles that make up the flexible, powerful midsection of your body called the core. On each side of your abs are your obliques, which help to support this central muscle mass. Every time you activate a large muscle group you also activate the core so that it can stabilise your body and provide a solid platform from which your strength can operate. During sport the core acts as an energy pipeline, transmitting the force you generate with one half of your body into the other – why else would you rotate your shoulders and arms just before you kick a football?

You can help to train your core for stability by replacing the weight bench you use for weightlifting with a gym ball (or Swiss ball), and by doing exercises such as shoulder presses and biceps curls while standing up. Having to stabilise yourself on a gym ball forces the muscles to work harder than they would if they were supported by a stable object such as a bench.

Rectus abdominis

The primary function of the rectus abdominis is trunk flexion, which is the movement you make when you're doing a crunch.

External obliques

The external obliques are the outermost abdominal muscles and are responsible for rotating your trunk.

Internal obliques

The second layer of muscle, which, like the external obliques, are used during trunk rotation.

Serratus anterior

The serratus anterior is found on the surface of the upper eight ribs at the side of your chest and pulls the scapula (shoulder blade) forward when you throw a punch.

Transverse abdominis

The transverse abdominis is the deepest lying of the abdominal muscles and is used to help compress the ribs.

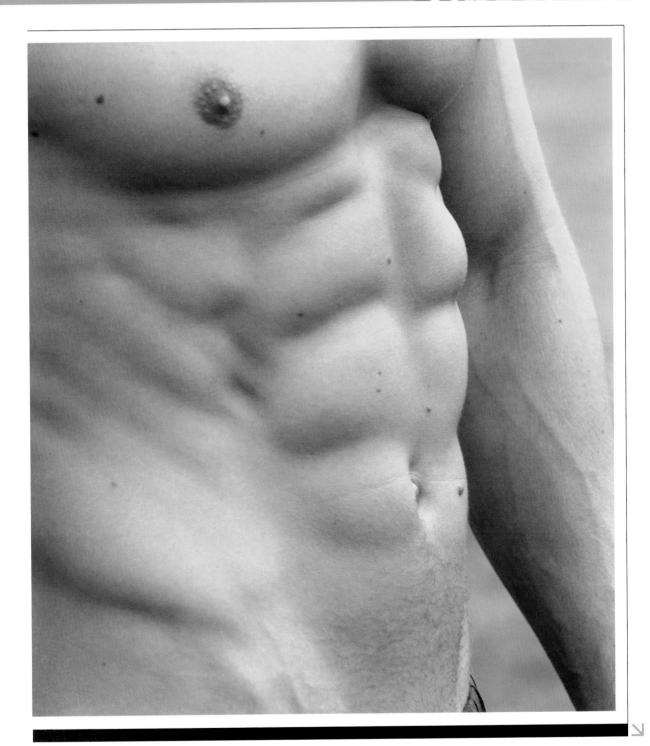

The abs classics

A small selection of the best six-pack-sculpting moves

When building a rock-solid stomach, there are a few simple rules you need to follow. First, you need to do a full-body workout several times a week. This will burn fat from around your midriff and build muscle all over your body, including your abs. Second, you need to do exercises that hit your upper abdominals, lower abdominals and obliques (side abs). That means doing three different abs exercises in each session. Third, you need to make your abs exercises harder over time. If you simply do the same exercise again and again, your body will become accustomed to it and stop building new muscle.

At the end of your full-body workout, try the exercises from this selection. Pick one that hits your upper abdominals, one that targets your lower abs and one for your obliques. Start with the basic exercises and build up to the tougher ones after a few weeks.

Make slow, controlled movements for each exercise, and concentrate on squeezing your abs for the maximum contraction. If you find that you get bored of doing these moves, don't worry, we've got lots of new exercises for you to try later in the book.

UPPER ABS

BASIC	A BIT TOUGHER	TOUGHER STILL	ADVANCED
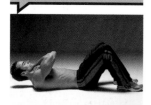	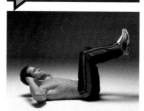	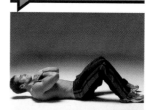	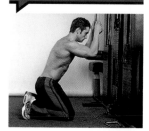
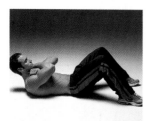	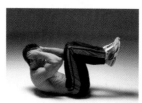	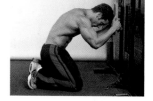	

Crunch
- Curl shoulders off the floor
- Hold at the top of the move
- Feet flat on floor

Tuck and crunch
- Thighs vertical
- Hands touching sides of head
- Curl torso forward while bringing knees back to meet elbows

Weight plate crunch
- Feet flat on floor
- Hold weight plate against your chest
- Curl torso towards knees
- Choose a weight that lets you complete 12–15 reps

High pulley crunch
- Grip rope handle in front of your face
- Curl ribcage towards pelvis
- Choose a weight that lets you do 12–15 reps

LOWER ABS

BASIC	A BIT TOUGHER	TOUGHER STILL	ADVANCED

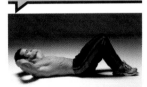
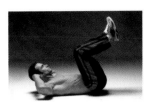

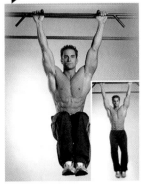

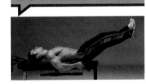
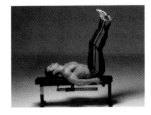

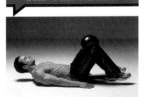
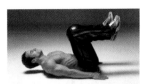

Reverse crunch
■ Knees bent at 90˚
■ Hands touching sides of head
■ Curl knees towards your chest

Hanging knee raise
■ Bring knees up as high as you can
■ Don't swing back and forth
■ Lower your feet as slowly as you can

Seated leg raise
■ Hold legs at around 45˚
■ Grip bench for support
■ Raise legs until your heels point at the ceiling, then lower them slowly

Medicine ball reverse curl
■ Knees bent at 90˚, gripping a medicine ball
■ Curl knees towards your chest
■ Do 12–15 reps

OBLIQUES

BASIC	A BIT TOUGHER	TOUGHER STILL	ADVANCED

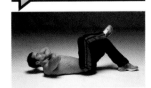
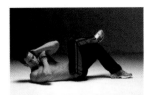

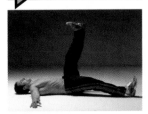
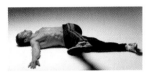

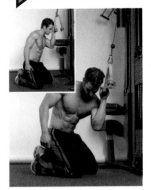

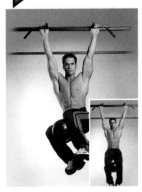

Crossover twist crunch
■ One hand touching side of head
■ Curl elbow towards opposite knee
■ Repeat on other side

Single leg over
■ Leg vertical
■ Arms out to sides
■ Twist torso to the side as far as you can go, and return
■ Repeat on the other side

One-arm pull-down crunch
■ Kneel face-on to the stack, knees pointing slightly to the side, and grip rope handle in one hand by your head
■ Curl ribcage towards pelvis
■ Do 12–15 reps on each side

Hanging medicine ball twist
■ Grip a medicine ball between your knees
■ Raise your knees up and to the side
■ Alternate sides each rep
■ Control the movement – don't swing

The abs rules

Follow these tips for a chiselled six-pack

1 DON'T DO SIT-UPS

There is no single best move for building a solid six-pack, least of all the simple sit-up as wedging your feet under a bench and raising your chest to your knees mainly works the hip flexors, not the abdominals.

2 Work your whole body

Compound exercises, such as squats and deadlifts, require the abs to provide stability throughout the move, so performing them as part of your training will stimulate both the deep-lying and outer core muscles to build a strong and stable midsection.

3 Hit your abs from all angles

Standard crunches will only hit the top part of your abs, but adding reverse crunches will work the bottom part, while twisting crunches will hit the obliques to help develop a complete six-pack.

4 KEEP CARDIO SHORT

Cardio exercise should revolve around interval and hill sessions rather than long, steady-paced runs to maximise calorie burn and help shift the layer of fat that will keep all your hard work hidden.

5 RING THE CHANGES

Variation is the key to keeping your abs working and developing. If you just repeat the same old routine and don't introduce any new exercises, your muscles will stop responding. Alternate your routines throughout the week to keep building abs.

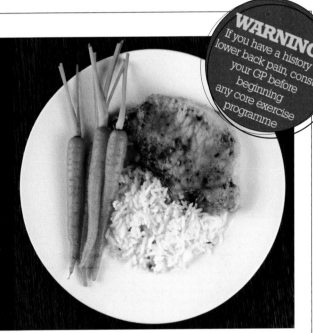

6 EAT MORE PROTEIN

To build muscle you need to eat between 1.5g and 2g of lean protein per kilo of bodyweight every day. Even then, you may not be able to see your six-pack if your body-fat percentage is higher than 10 per cent, so you need to burn more calories than you consume to shift that excess flab.

7 Train standing up

Doing all your abs and lower back exercise on a mat means that one side of your body is switched off when you're working the other. Standing exercises that involve a twit or rotation, such as a woodchop on the cable machine, work the core as a single unit to provide better protection against strains or injury.

8 Save the abs until last

Working your abs at the start of your session can fatigue them so that they don't provide the stability needed for big compound moves, meaning you'll have to settle for lifting less. Work your abs later in the session, or devote an entire workout to them.

9 TREAT THE ABS LIKE ANY OTHER MUSCLE

To build your abs work them like you would your other major muscle groups. Start with sets of 10 to 15 repetitions, leaving a day's rest between sessions, and increase the intensity by adding extra sets. Bashing out 200 reps of an abs exercise every day won't lead to a six-pack but a hernia.

10 GET DOWN LOWER

Defining the top four abdominals is easier than revealing the bottom two; unless you include specific exercises to work them hard. Start with reverse crunches, with your legs either on a Swiss ball or straight up in the air.

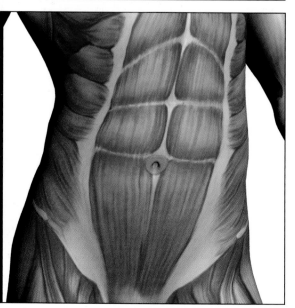

11 Do static holds

Muscles are made from both fast-twitch and slow-twitch fibres. Holding a weight in static position targets both groups at once, improving the muscle's overall strength and stability in one exercise. Moves such as the plank are most effective, providing you hold the position for more than five seconds.

12 Add resistance to crunches to build muscle

Start with a dumbbell or medicine ball across your chest and close to your body to add resistance to crunches and force your abs to work harder. Gradually increase the difficulty by extending your arms above your head, holding the weight up.

13 HAVE PERFECT POSTURE

Maintaining good posture throughout the day, even when you're sitting at your desk, will activate those all-important deep-lying stabilising muscles that are vital for a strong core. So sit up straight!

14 BUILD IT UP

Don't get too comfortable with your abs-building routine – if you're breezing through the exercises then try increasing the resistance. Gradually adding heavier weights into your training will help to keep those muscles getting stronger.

15 | DON'T IGNORE THE DEEP-LYING MUSCLES

Performing exercises such as the plank work the inner core muscles that provide the stability that allows the outer muscles to become stronger and bigger.

16 Stretch your core

Improving your core flexibility aids recovery. Long, supple muscles allow for better blood flow which helps nutrients to reach your muscles.

17 Slow down your reps

Muscles will only grow if they are held under tension, and slowing down the speed of each rep will keep them engaged for longer. For crunches, count to three on the way up, hold for two, before lowering again in three.

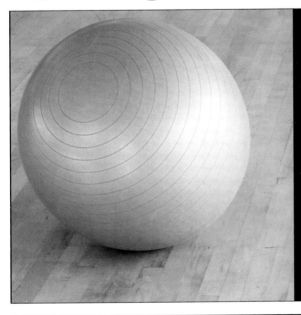

18 USE A GYM BALL

Training on an unstable surface, such as a gym ball, recruits far more muscle fibres to hold you steady than on a flat environment. All these fibres receive microscopic tears, which are repaired and so grow back bigger and stronger.

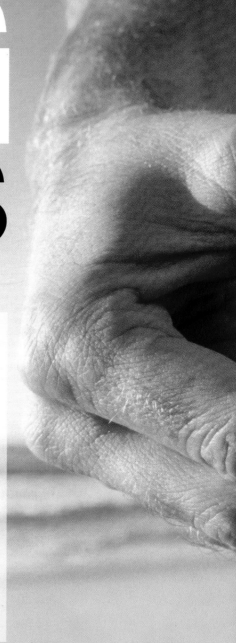

BIG FAT LIES

Separate fact from fiction with the truth behind common abs myths

 You can target areas for fat loss
It is impossible to strip fat from your belly by doing countless sit-ups and crunches. Any fat burned through exercise will be taken from stores all over the body. Men tend to store excess body fat around the belly, whereas women are more likely to be bigger around the hips and thighs.

 Sit-ups are great for fat-burning
Abs exercises are not great calorie burners as they target just one muscle group. Burning just one pound of fat would require 250,000 crunches, or two weeks of non-stop crunching!

 Crunches are good for your back
Crunches are one of the best abs-building exercises out there, but they do little for the back muscles that work with the abs to provide functional strength. Crunches strengthen the midsection as they force the muscles to shorten, but equally strong back muscles are vital for lengthening the muscle to offer a good range of motion and provide muscular balance.

 You should always work the abs while lying down
The abs are designed to help you rotate your torso at the waist or prevent it from rotating when you don't want it to. Standing up during your abs routine allows the muscles to work in a more natural way to improve balance, endurance and control, while also working your shoulders and traps.

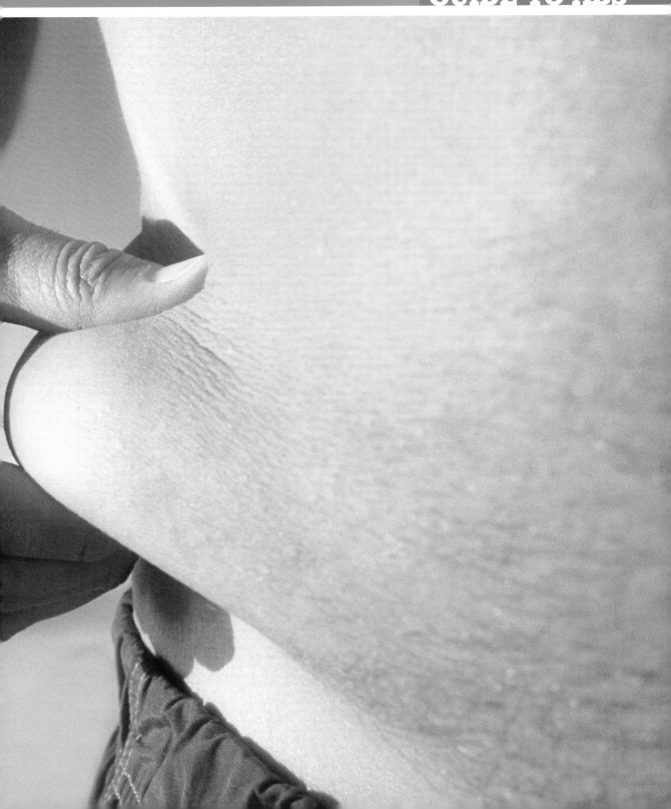

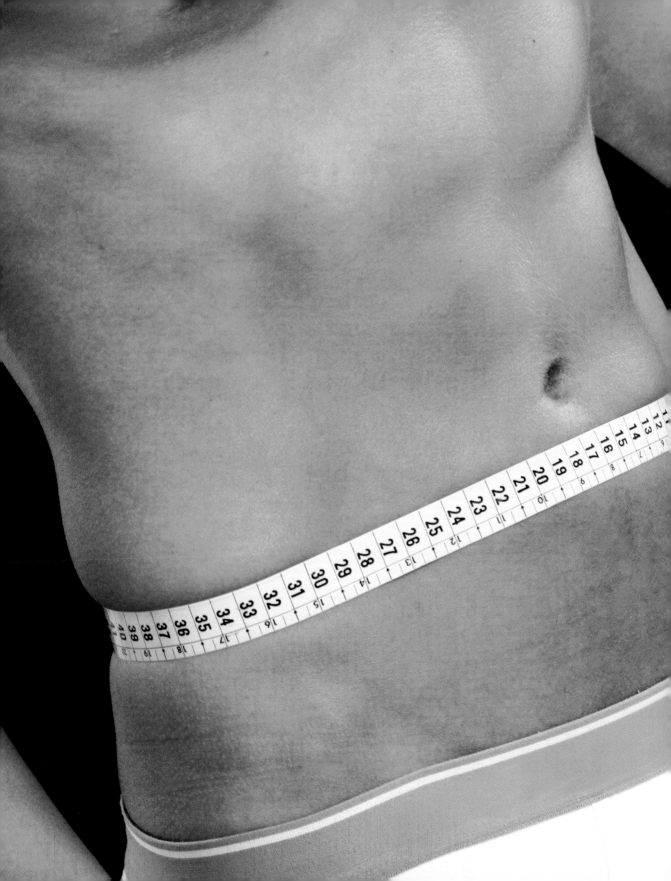

'**Burning one pound of fat would require 250,000 crunches, or two weeks of non-stop crunching**'

MYTH Sucking in your waist makes your core stronger

To build a spine-protecting muscle belt while working your whole abdominals section, you shouldn't suck your waist in while performing exercise but push it out, as if you were straining for a bowel movement. Nice. But this will create the type of abdominal strength that stabilises and protects the spine when doing heavy squats and deadlifts.

MYTH Functional exercises don't build big abs

Of course a six-pack looks great, but the real benefits of a solid midsection are a strong and healthier back and improved sports performance. Including functional exercises that require the abs to perform as they would during sports and other physical activity will help build a more balanced – and noticeable – stomach.

MYTH You should work your abs every day

The abs are a muscle group all of their own, just like the back and chest, so they need to be rested after a session so that they can recover and grow back stronger. Overtraining of the abs is a common reason why muscle gains plateau.

MYTH Always start with your upper abs

The lower abdominals are often weaker than the upper abs and obliques because they are not used as frequently. The upper region also has a role in stabilising the torso during lower abs training, so it's important that these muscles are fresh and strong when doing specific lower abs work. Try shaking up the training order once your lower abs are as strong as the rest of the midsection.

MYTH The abdominal region is a single muscle

The abs are a collection of muscles including the rectus abdominis, transverse abdominis and the internal and external obliques. These muscles cannot be completely isolated during exercise. However, twisting the torso will work the obliques, crunching your upper and lower body targets the upper abs, or bringing your legs up to your body stimulates the lower region.

MYTH Performing dozens of reps aids abs definition

Muscle shape is determined exclusively by genetics, so no amount of exercise will change their shape. But you can increase muscle mass by performing sets of low-rep, high-resistance moves.

The anatomy of

Master the basics for effective sit-ups with this form guide

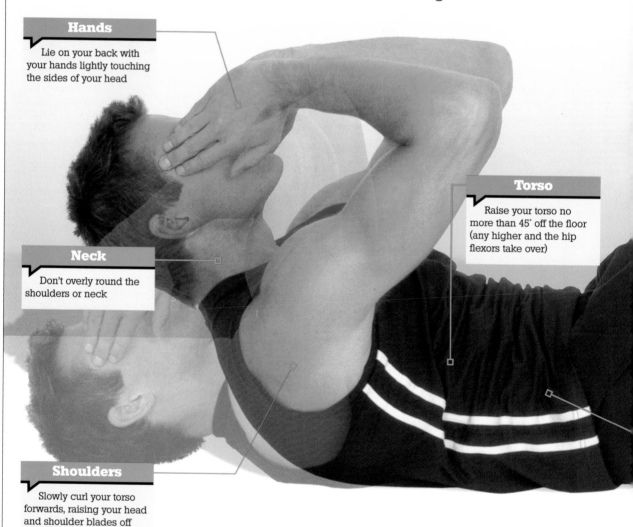

Hands

Lie on your back with your hands lightly touching the sides of your head

Torso

Raise your torso no more than 45° off the floor (any higher and the hip flexors take over)

Neck

Don't overly round the shoulders or neck

Shoulders

Slowly curl your torso forwards, raising your head and shoulder blades off the floor

the crunch

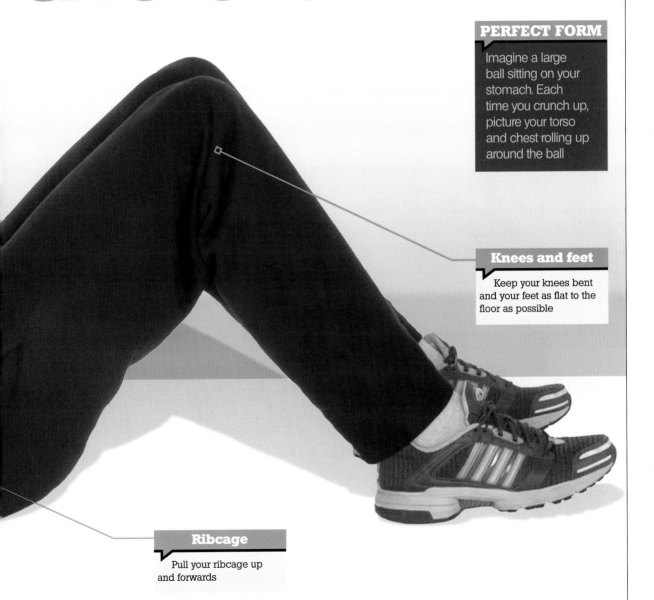

PERFECT FORM

Imagine a large ball sitting on your stomach. Each time you crunch up, picture your torso and chest rolling up around the ball

Knees and feet

Keep your knees bent and your feet as flat to the floor as possible

Ribcage

Pull your ribcage up and forwards

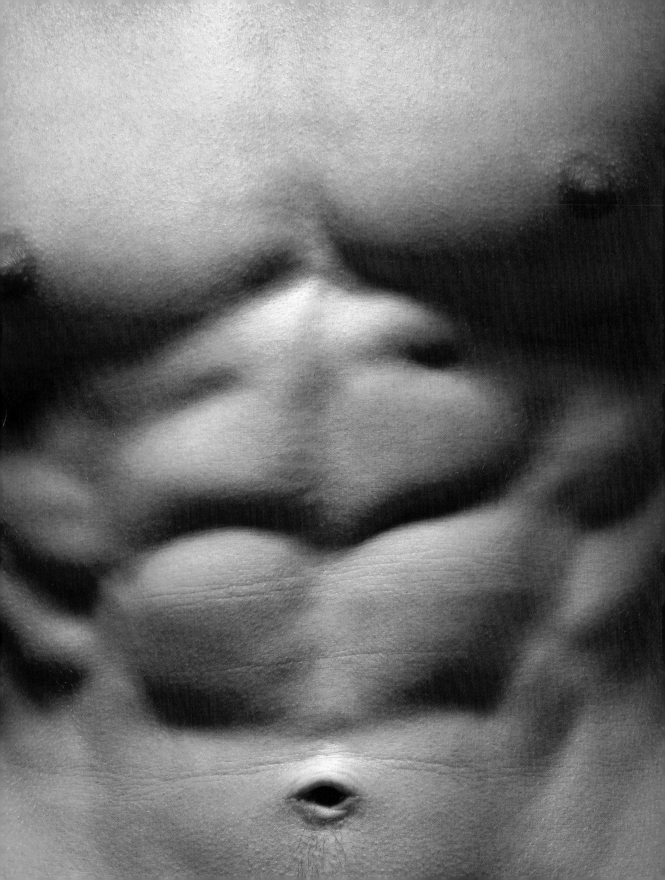

The 72 best abs exercises

You'll never run out of ways to build a six-pack with this selection of moves

We know you want to build an impressive six-pack – that's why you're reading this book. We also know that simply doing crunches won't get you that six-pack. If you just do one move all the time, your muscles adapt to its demands and your growth will plateau. You need to hit your abdominal muscles in a variety of ways and from all angles to keep them stimulated. This is the way to get the hard abs you hanker after – and it'll stop you getting bored with endless crunches as well.

Most of the 72 exercises we've collected here can be done using simple equipment such as a gym ball or a set of dumb-bells, so you may not even have to leave the house to work your abs. We've rated them on a three-level scale from 'easy' to 'hard', but you can make any of the weights exercises harder by adding more weight or an unstable platform such as a gym or Bosu ball.

There are also warm-up and warm-down tips, so turn the page for our anthology of abs exercises and get to work on that six-pack.

TURN OVER TO BEGIN YOUR MOVES

Warm-up

Prepare your muscles before every workout with this routine

Doing a warm-up before your workout can seem like valuable time wasted, but it's well worth spending ten or 15 minutes warming up rather than wasting days laid up at home with damaged muscles or ligaments.

The purpose of a warm-up is simple: to raise your core temperature and prepare your muscles for the work to come. By doing some light cardiovascular exercise – such as running, cycling or rowing – you make your heart beat faster, which pumps oxygen and nutrients to your muscles and elevates your body's temperature. Warm muscles are more elastic, so you can work them through a greater range of motion with less risk of injury.

Once you've done the cardio warm-up, you should move on to targeting the muscles directly with dynamic stretches. These will help to increase the temperature of your muscles yet further, stretch them gently and get them ready for heavy lifting. Dynamic stretches differ from static stretches (see p78) because you are moving continuously and placing the muscle under increased tension with each repetition, preparing it for the training you're about to perform.

Once you begin your workout it makes sense to do your first set of each lift with a light weight, so that you further prepare the specific muscles and tendons you are targeting for heavier weights in the following sets.

Warm-up: Cardio

■ **Begin with ten minutes of gentle cardio such as cross-training, running, cycling or rowing. By the end you should** be sweating gently and puffing, but not out of breath. You don't want to burn out before your workout begins!

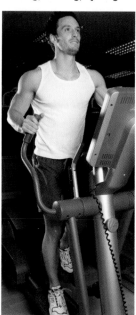
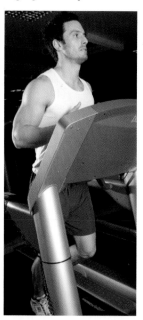
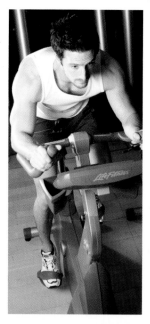
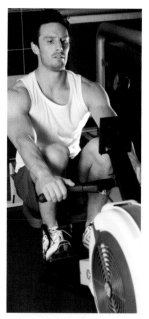

Warm-up: Dynamic stretches

Do ten repetitions of each of the following exercises, alternating sides with each rep where appropriate. Start gently and aim to increase the range of motion with each rep.

1 Lunge with reverse flye

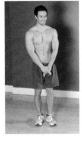
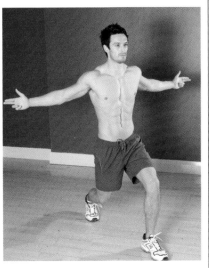

■ Spread your arms wide

■ Step forward and bend your knees

2 Lateral lunge with twist

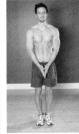
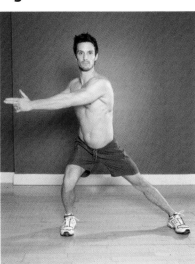

■ Step to the side and bend your knees

■ Rotate your body to the side

3 Alternating split deadlift

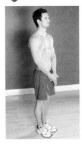
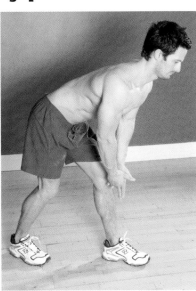

■ Step forward and lean over from the hips

■ Feel the stretch in your hamstrings

4 Squat-to-overhead reach

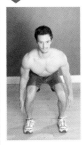
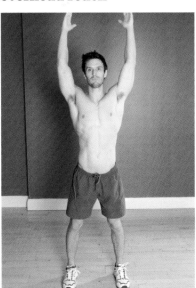

■ Squat down with your back straight

■ Stand up and raise your arms

No **kit**

Exercises you can do anywhere, any time

EASY

1 **Crunch**
Target: upper abs
A | Feet flat on floor
B | Curl shoulders off floor, keeping lower back in contact with mat
C | Pause at the top and lower slowly to the start

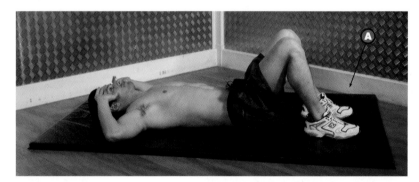

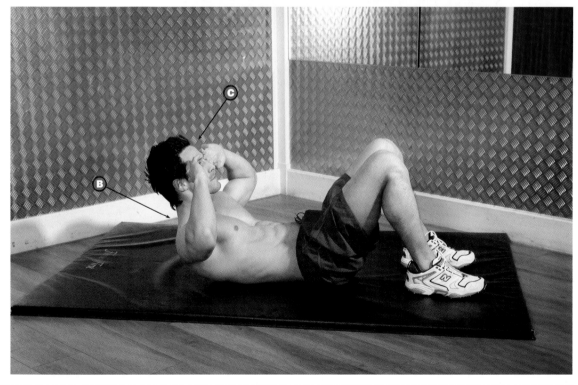

2 ▶ Plank

Target: whole core

A | Elbows directly beneath shoulders

B | Body in a straight line from head to heels

C | Hold the position for as long as you can

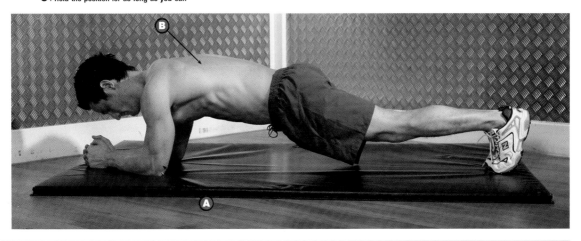

3 ▶ Reverse crunch

Target: lower abs

A | Start with thighs vertical and knees bent at 90°

B | Lift hips off floor and curl knees towards chest

C | Pause at top and lower slowly to the start

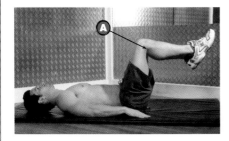

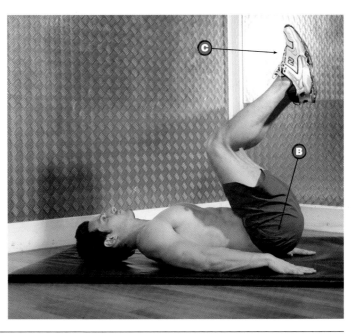

4 Lying crisscross

Target: lower abs

A | Place hands under backside for stability

B | Hold feet 10cm or so off floor with straight legs

C | Cross feet over and under for as long as you can manage

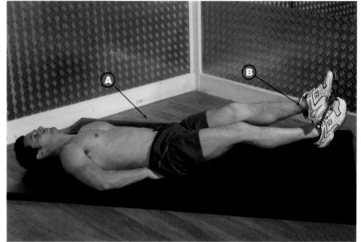

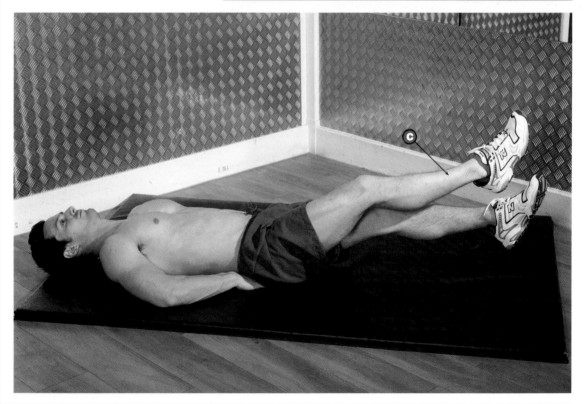

72 ABS MOVES

5 Crossover twist crunch

Target: side abs

A | Place one foot on opposite knee

B | Curl shoulders off floor and twist body so elbow touches knee

C | Pause at top and lower slowly, then repeat on opposite side

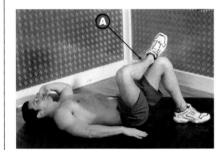

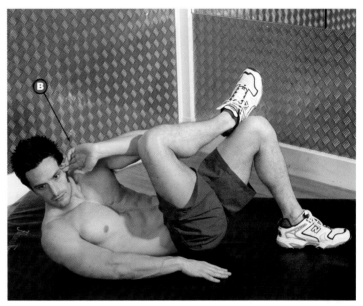

6 Side plank

Target: side abs

A | Elbow directly beneath shoulder

B | Body in a straight line from head to feet

C | Hold position for as long as you can

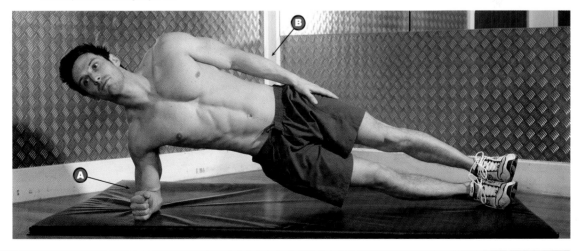

MEDIUM

7 | Legs up crunch

Target: upper abs

A | Thighs vertical and knees bent at 90°

B | Curl shoulders off floor

C | Pause at top and lower slowly to the start

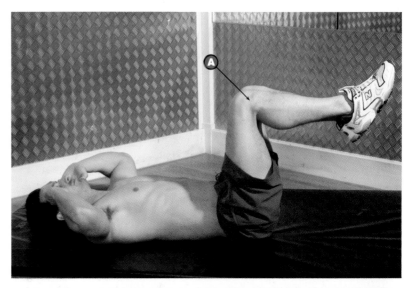

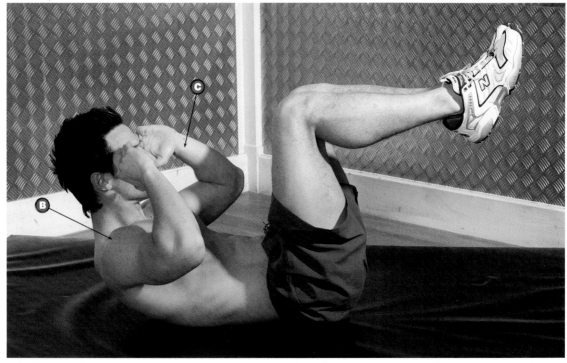

8 Two-point box

Target: whole core

A | Start on all fours

B | Raise opposing arm and leg straight out

C | Pause at top, lower slowly to the start and repeat on other side

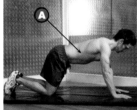

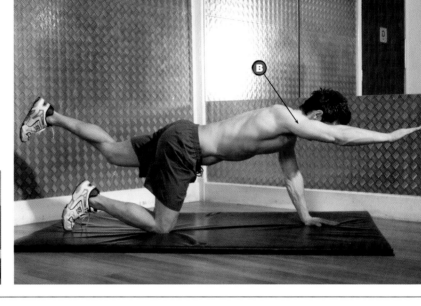

9 Leg lower

Target: lower abs

A | Start with legs pointing straight up

B | Place hands under backside for support

C | Lower legs slowly to just above floor and return to the start

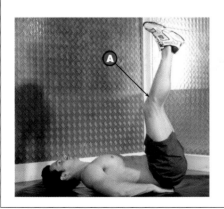

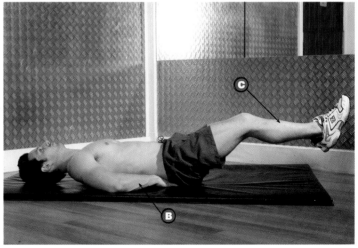

MEDIUM

10 ▶ Hip raise

Target: lower abs

A | Start with legs pointing straight up

B | Lift hips off floor and push feet towards ceiling

C | Hold for a second and then lower slowly to the start

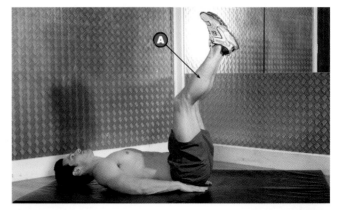

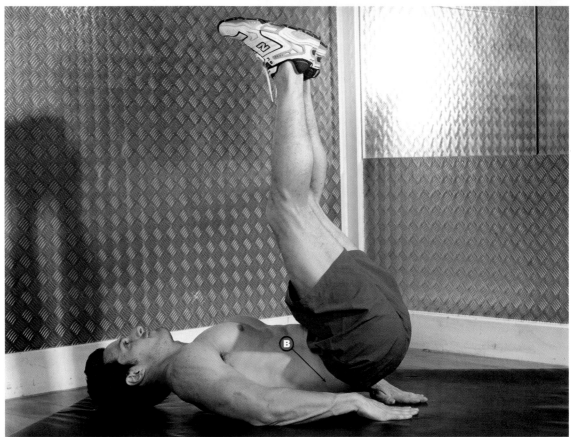

MEDIUM

11 ▶ Side crunch
Target: side abs

A I Lie on your side with upper hand touching temple
B I Curl torso upwards as far as you can
C I Pause at top and lower slowly back to the start

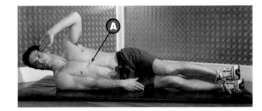

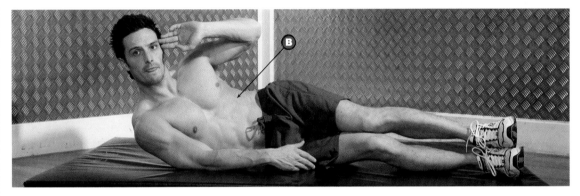

12 ▶ Single leg over
Target: side abs

A I Start with one leg pointing straight up
B I Hands out either side for support
C I Rotate lower body until foot is just above floor, then return

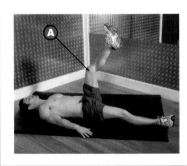

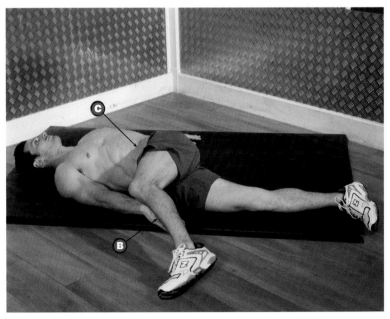

HARD

13 Jackknife

Target: upper and lower abs

A | Lie on your back with arms and legs held just off floor

B | Bring arms and legs up to meet above your stomach

C | Lower slowly to the start, keeping arms and legs straight

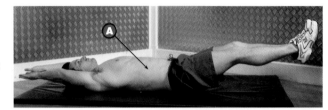

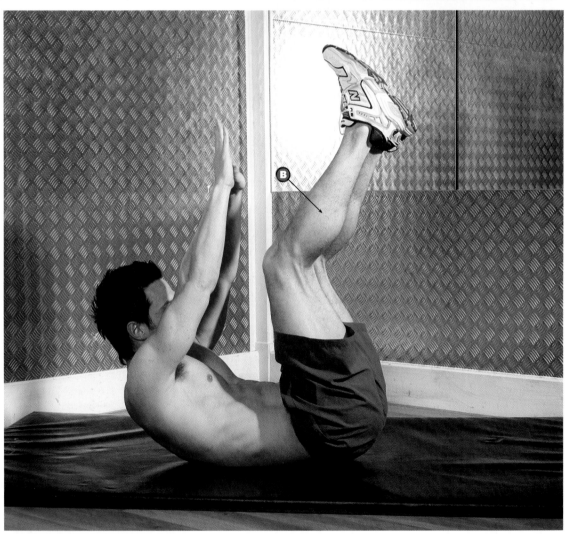

14 ▶ Long arm crunch

Target: upper abs

A | Hold arms straight out behind your head for extra leverage

B | Curl shoulders off floor, keeping arms in same position

C | Hold at top and then lower slowly to the start

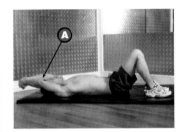

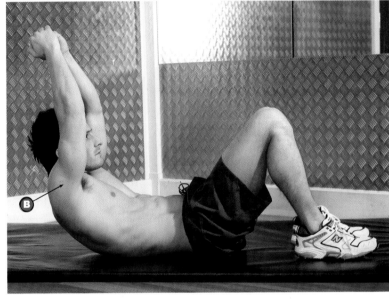

15 ▶ Cycling Russian twist

Target: whole core

A | Hold torso at around 45˚ to floor and lift feet off floor

B | Turn torso to left while drawing right knee in

C | Twist from side to side while cycling legs back and forth

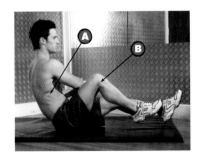

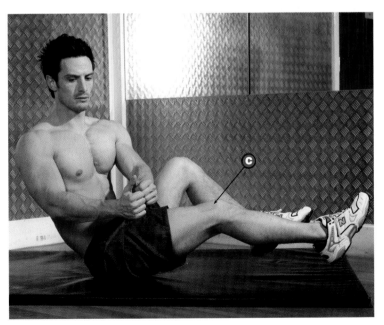

HARD

16 Modified V-sit

Target: upper and lower abs

A | Lie with feet held off floor and hands over your thighs

B | Sit up and bring your knees in to your chest

C | Lower slowly to the start and repeat

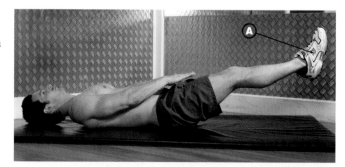

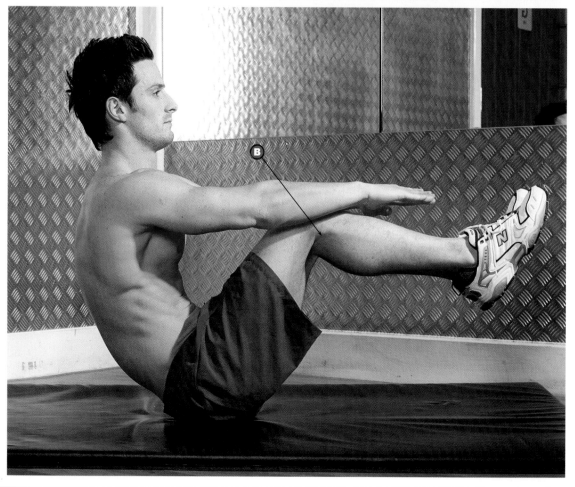

17 Raised side plank

Target: side abs

A | Elbow directly beneath shoulder

B | Hold body in a straight line and lift upper arm and leg

C | Hold position for as long as you can

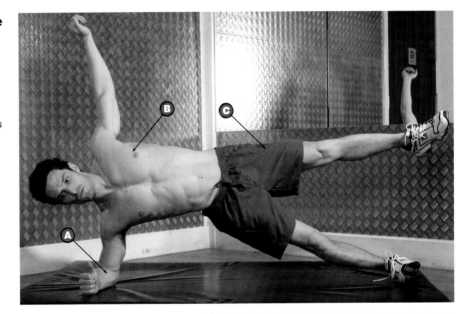

18 Double leg over

Target: side abs

A | Start with both legs pointing straight up

B | Arms out either side for support

C | Turn lower body to one side until feel are just off floor, then return

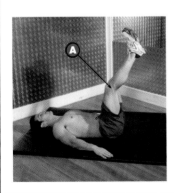

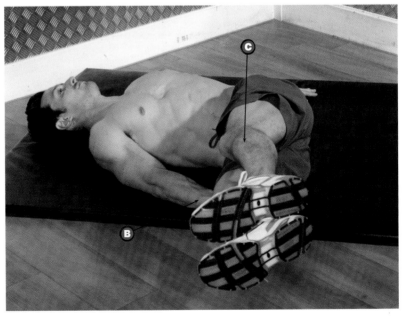

Dumb bells

Add some weight to make your abs work harder

EASY

19 ▸ Punch ups

Target: whole core

A | Hold a dumb-bell in each hand and stand with feet shoulder-width apart

B | Turn body to one side and perform uppercut

C | Twist powerfully from side to side, punching each side

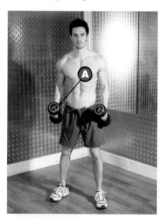

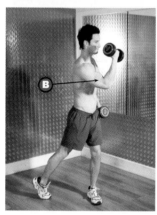

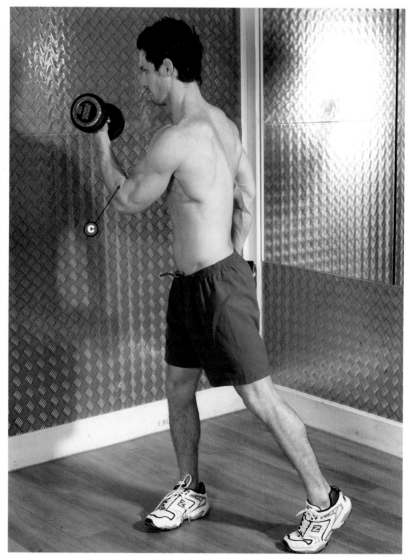

20 Weighted crunch

Target: upper abs

A | Hold dumb-bell across chest

B | Curl shoulders off floor, keeping lower back in contact with mat

C | Pause at top and then lower slowly to the start

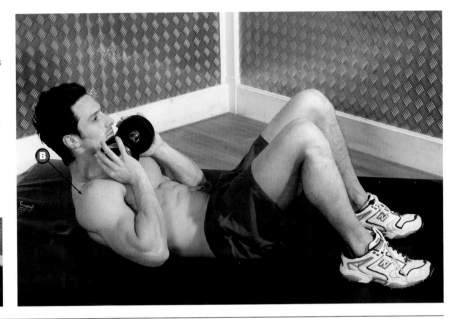

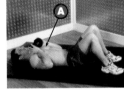

21 Punch-up crunch

Target: upper abs

A | Hold a dumb-bell in each hand

B | Curl shoulders off floor and punch straight out with one hand

C | Return slowly to the start and repeat with other hand on next rep

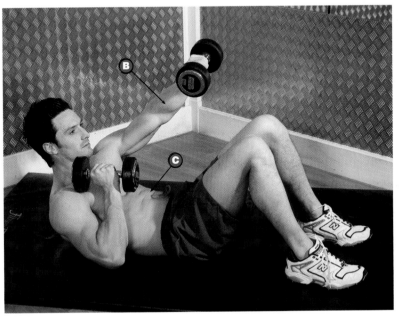

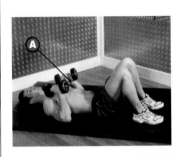

22 Russian twist

Target: side abs

A | Hold dumb-bell straight out in front of your chest

B | Turn torso around to one side

C | Twist powerfully from side to side, keeping your back upright

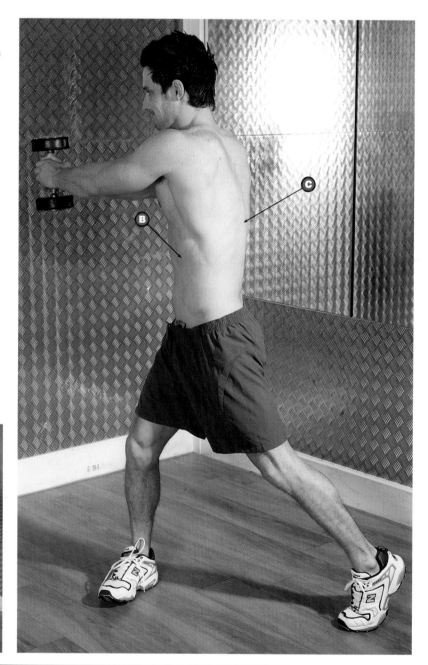

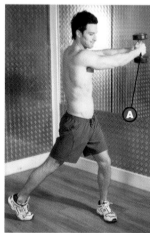

HARD

23 Weighted corkscrew

Target: lower abs

A | Grasp dumb-bell between your feet and hold legs vertical

B | Lift hips off floor and push feet towards ceiling

C | At top twist to one side, lower and repeat to other side

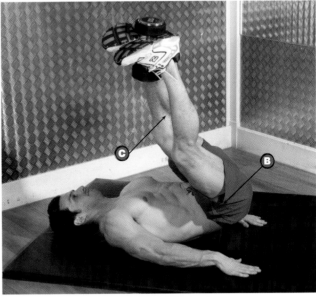

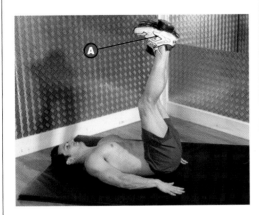

24 Woodchop

Target: whole core

A | Hold dumb-bell in both hands and stand with feet shoulder-width apart

B | Bring weight down to outside of thigh, keeping your back straight

C | Twist torso and bring weight up over opposite shoulder

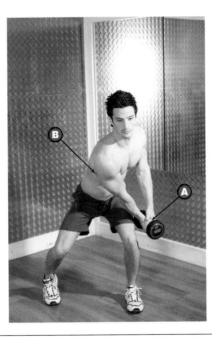

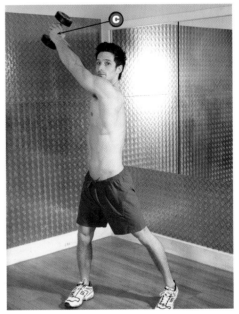

Gym **ball**

Keep your abs and core muscles tensed to hold the ball steady

EASY

25 ▶ Gym ball crunch

Target: upper abs

A | With ball beneath lower back, lie back as far as you can
B | Curl shoulders up, keeping lower back on ball
C | Pause at top, then lower slowly to the start

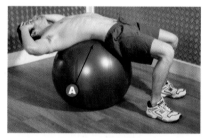

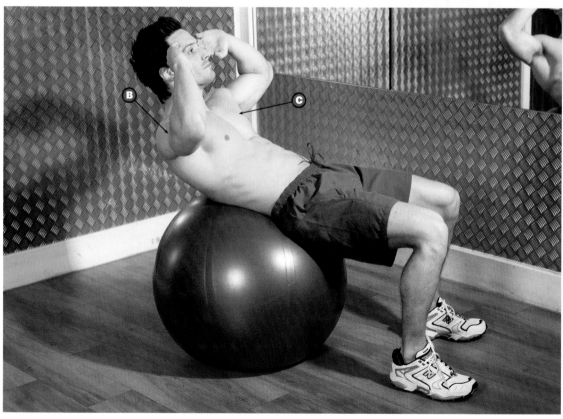

MEDIUM

26 Gym ball reverse crunch

Target: lower abs

A | Hold ball between your calves and the backs of your thighs

B | Curl hips off floor and bring knees towards chest

C | Pause at top, then lower slowly to the start

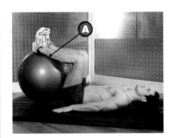

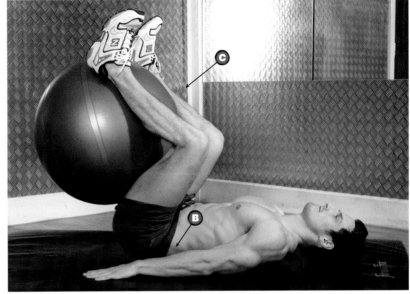

27 Gym ball twist curl

Target: side abs

A | With ball beneath lower back, lie back as far as you can

B | Curl shoulders up and twist torso to one side

C | Lower slowly to the start and repeat to other side

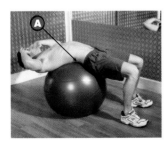

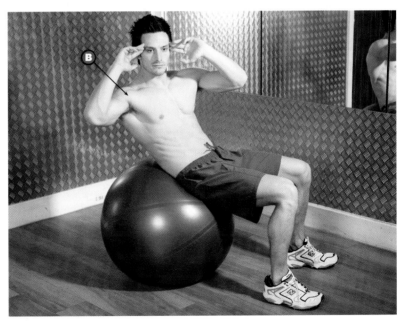

28 Gym ball jackknife

Target: upper abs

A | Hold body in a straight line with feet on ball and hands under shoulders

B | Draw your knees in towards your chest

C | Return to the start without letting your hips sag

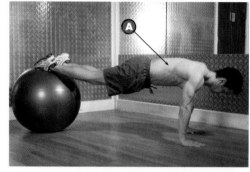

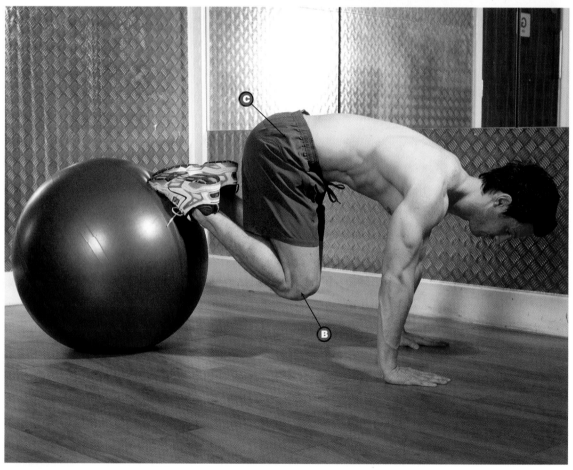

MEDIUM

29 Gym ball rollout

Target: lower abs

A | Kneel and place forearms on top of ball

B | Roll ball away from you as far as you can, holding your body steady

C | Return slowly, keeping your back flat at all times

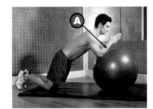

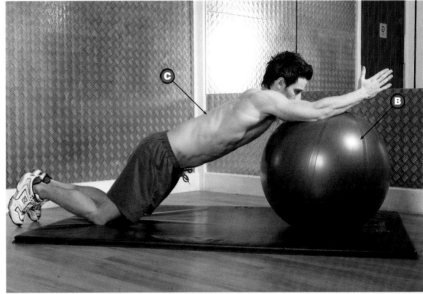

30 Gym ball leg scissors

Target: side abs

A | Hold ball off floor between your feet

B | Rotate lower body to one side

C | Rotate to other side and repeat back and forth

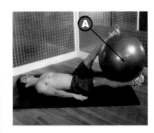

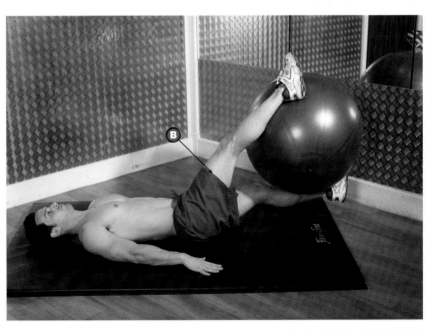

MEDIUM

31 **Gym ball lateral crunch**

Target: side abs

A | Lie side-on to ball and jam your feet against wall for support

B | Lift torso sideways as far as you can

C | Pause at top and lower slowly, then repeat on other side

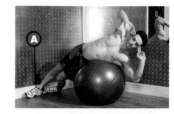

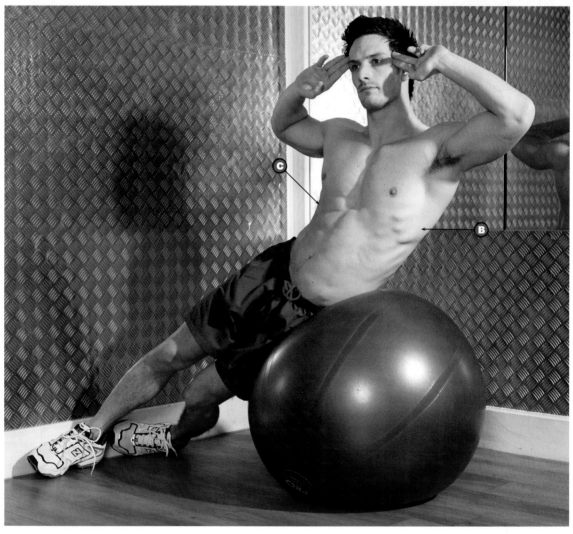

MEDIUM

32 Gym ball plank

Target: whole core

A | Rest weight on elbows on ball

B | Hold your body in a straight line from head to heels

C | Maintain position for as long as you can

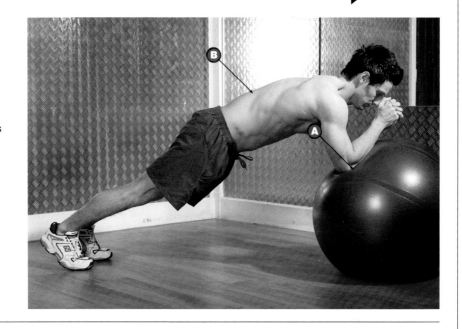

33 Gym ball dumb-bell pullover

Target: whole core

A | Lie back on ball and hold dumb-bell behind head with straight arms

B | Keep body straight from head to knees

C | Pull dumb-bell over chest, keeping arms straight

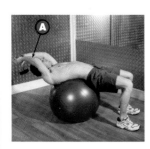

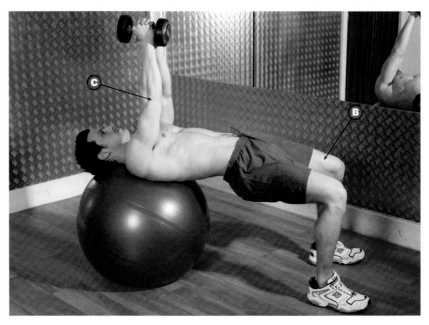

HARD

34 Gym ball side plank

Target: side abs

A | Rest one elbow on ball

B | Hold body in a straight line from head to feet

C | Maintain position for as long as you can

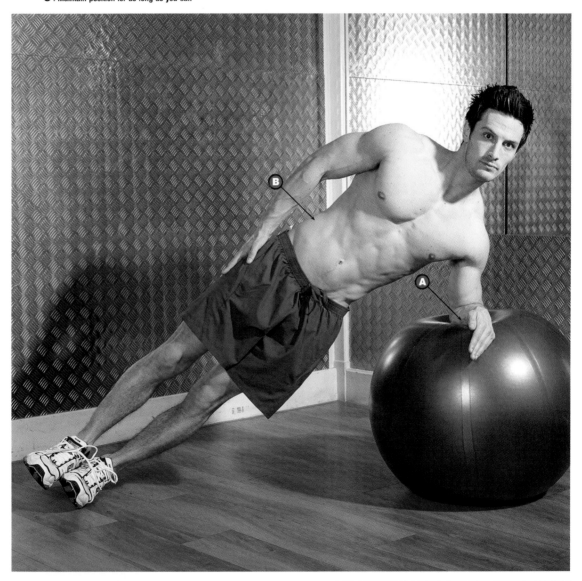

35 Gym ball passing V-sit

Target: upper and lower abs

A | Hold ball between your feet, keeping arms and legs straight
B | Lift legs and arms together to pass the ball from feet to hands
C | Lower arms and legs slowly, then pass ball back and forth

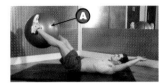
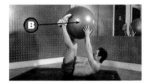

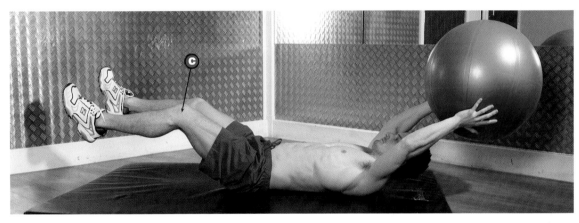

36 Scorpions

Target: whole core

A | Get into press-up position with one foot on ball
B | Bend other knee and twist body to one side
C | Twist body to other side, bringing knee underneath you

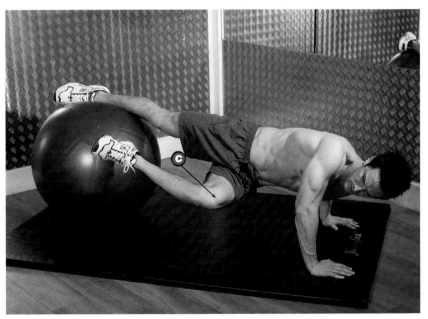

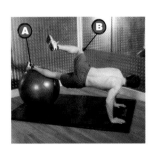

Gym ball & **dumb-bells**

Pair weight with wobble for a double hit on your abs

37 | Weighted gym ball crunch

Target: upper abs

A | Hold weight across chest

B | Lie back as far as you can with ball beneath lower back

C | Curl shoulders up without lifting lower back off ball

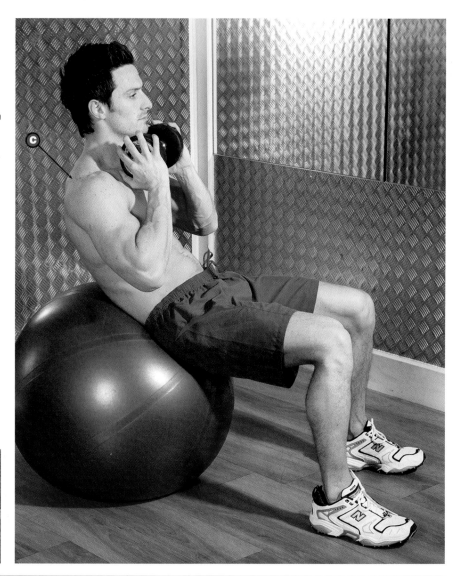

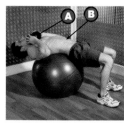

MEDIUM

38 Gym ball crunch to press

Target: upper abs

A | Hold a dumb-bell in each hand and lie back on ball

B | Curl shoulders up and press weights away from you at top

C | Pause at top and lower slowly to the start

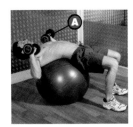

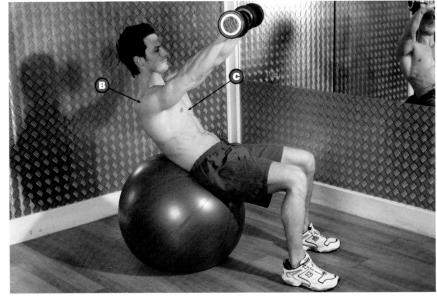

39 Gym ball dumb-bell row

Target: whole core

A | Lie with ball beneath your abdomen

B | Hold body in a straight line with weights hanging down

C | Draw weights up to sides and squeeze shoulder blades together

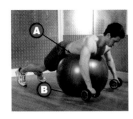

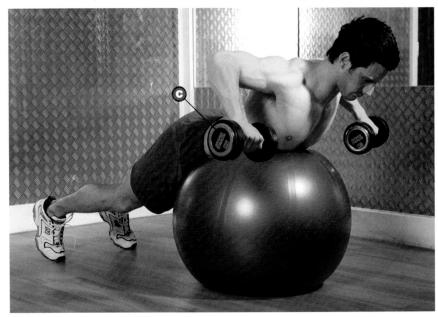

MEDIUM

40 Gym ball Russian twist

Target: side abs

A | Rest head and shoulders on ball and hold dumb-bell straight up

B | Keep body straight from head to knees

C | Rotate upper body from side to side while keeping arms straight

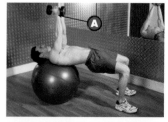

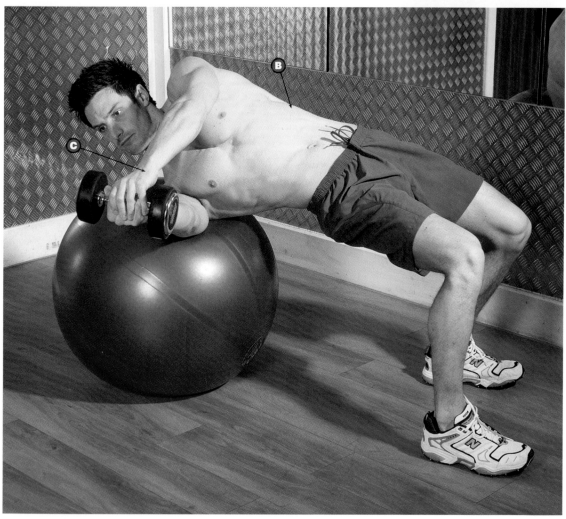

HARD

41 ▶ Gym ball overhead crunch

Target: upper abs

A | Lie back on ball and hold dumb-bell out behind head

B | Curl shoulders up, keeping arms in the same position

C | Pause at top and lower slowly to the start

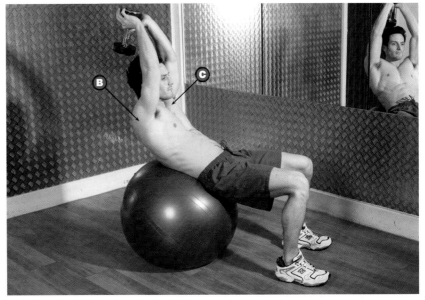
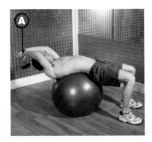

42 ▶ Gym ball side plank with lateral raise

Target: side abs

A | Rest elbow on ball and hold body in a straight line

B | With straight arm, raise weight until level with shoulders

C | Hold position while raising and lowering weight slowly

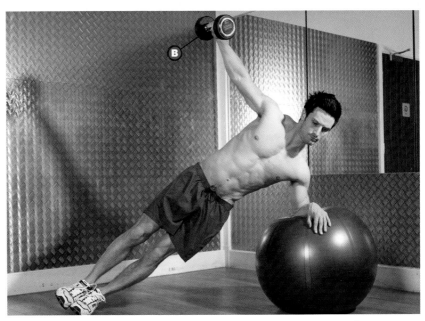
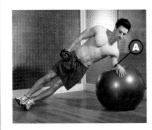

Medicine **ball**

Explosive moves with a heavy ball add an extra dimension to your abs

EASY

43 **One-leg slam-down**

Target: upper abs

A | Stand on one leg and hold ball over head

B | Bring down ball powerfully and throw it to floor

C | Keep core strong throughout move

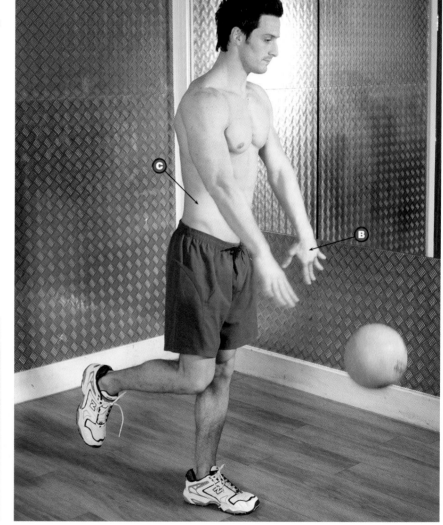

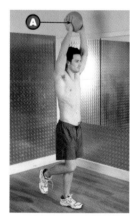

44 One-leg overhead toss

Target: whole core

A | Stand on one leg and hold ball over head

B | Toss ball from hand to hand

C | Keep body steady and upright throughout move

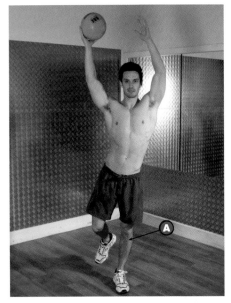
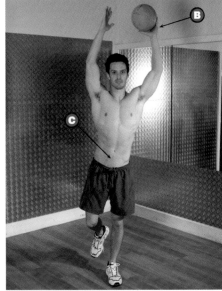

45 Standing throw

Target: side abs

A | Stand in split stance, one foot in front of other

B | Bring ball back over one shoulder, turning torso to that side

C | Twist body powerfully and throw ball against wall or to partner

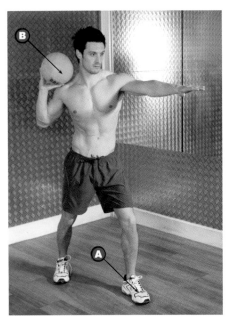
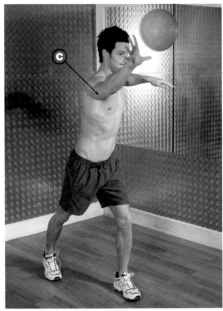

MEDIUM

46 Medicine ball pullover crunch

Target: upper abs

A | Lie with ball held straight out behind head
B | Lift shoulders and back off floor
C | Bring ball down hard in front of you

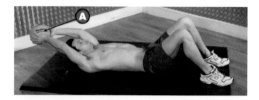

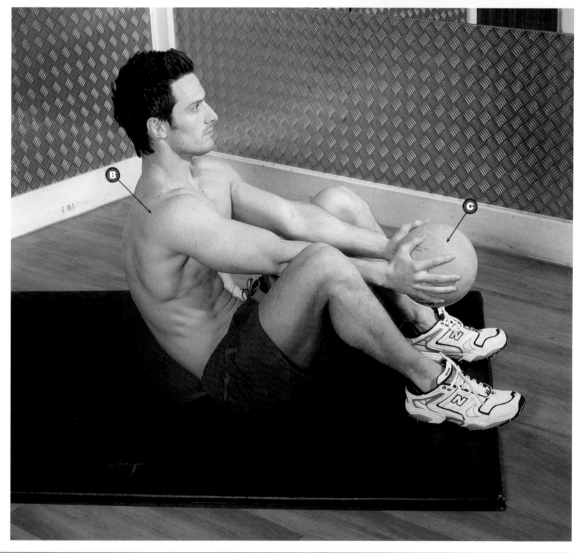

47 Medicine ball reverse crunch

Target: lower abs

A | Hold ball between your knees with thighs vertical

B | Curl knees towards chest, lifting hips off floor

C | Pause at top and lower slowly to the start

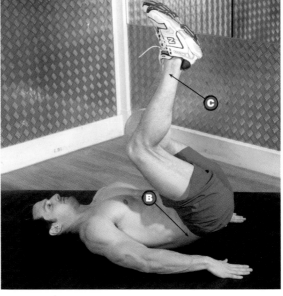

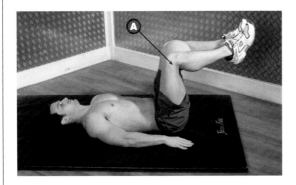

48 Side throws

Target: side abs

A | Hold ball with straight arms in front of chest

B | Twist torso to one side

C | Twist powerfully to other side and throw ball to partner

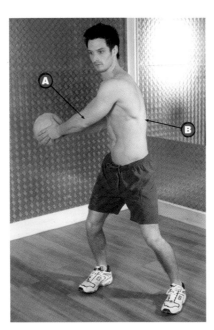

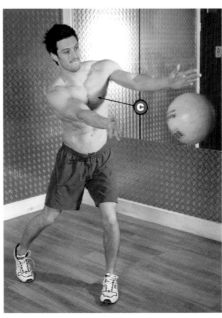

49 Medicine ball round body pass

Target: whole core

A | Sit with body leaning back and feet held off the floor
B | Maintain position while moving ball around your body
C | Reverse direction of ball from time to time

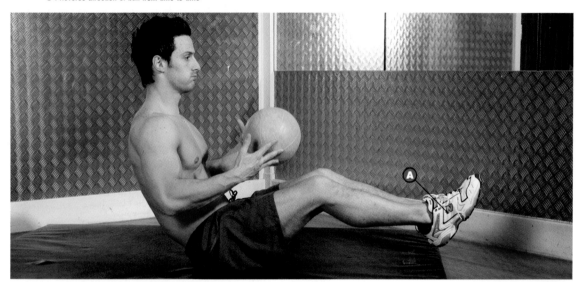

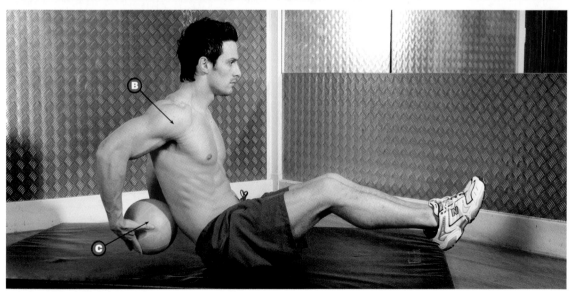

HARD

50 Crunch throw

Target: upper abs
A | Hold ball against chest
B | Curl shoulders off floor powerfully and throw ball to partner
C | Catch return throw and return slowly to the start

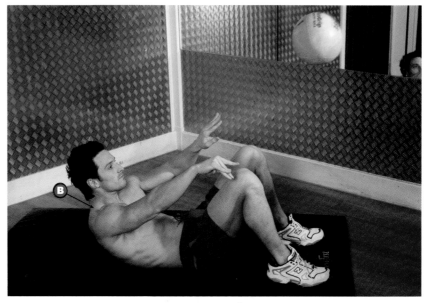

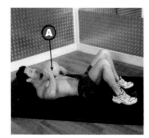

51 Medicine ball sledgehammer

Target: whole core
A | Stand with feet apart and hold ball over head
B | Bring ball down powerfully to between your knees and return
C | Keep your back straight and core muscles tensed throughout

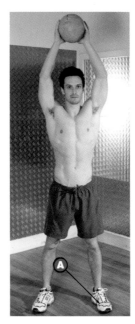

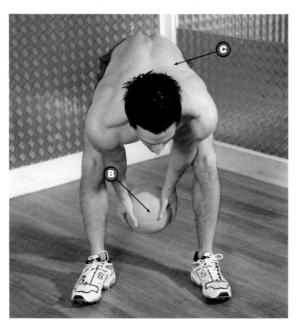

52 | Medicine ball leg drops

Target: lower abs

A | Grasp ball between your feet and hold legs straight up

B | Slowly lower your legs until feet are just above floor

C | Return to the start and repeat

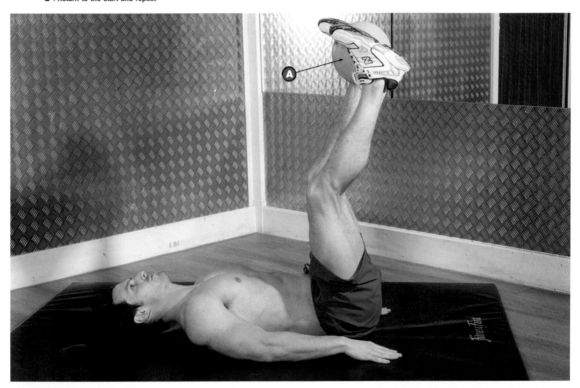

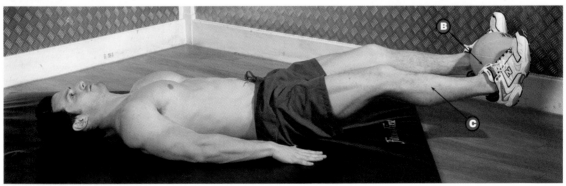

53 Medicine ball seated Russian twist

Target: side abs

A | Sit leaning at about 45° to floor, keeping your back straight and knees bent

B | Hold ball with straight arms and twist torso to one side

C | Twist from side to side, keeping your back straight throughout

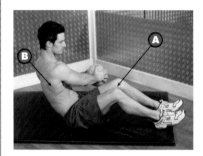

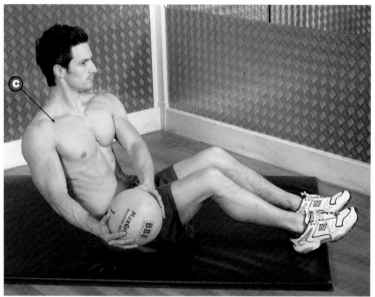

54 Medicine ball lunge woodchop

Target: whole core

A | Stand straight and lift ball over one shoulder

B | Step forward and lower into lunge with front knee over front foot

C | Chop ball down and across body, keeping your back straight

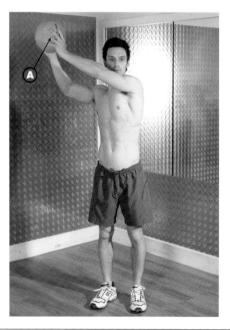

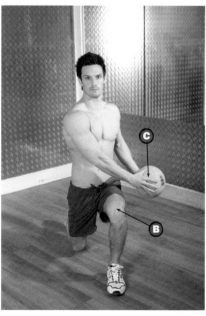

Cable

The cable machine ensures constant resistance throughout each move

EASY

55 **High cable crunch**
Target: upper abs
A | Kneel before a high cable and hold handle in front of face
B | Tense abs and curl shoulders down, keeping hands in same place
C | Pause at bottom and rise slowly to the start

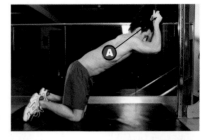

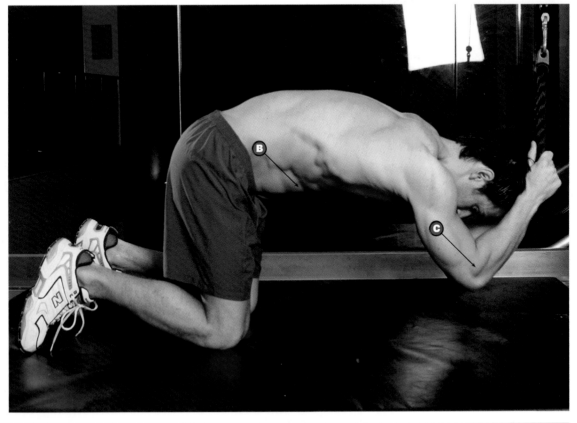

56 One-arm row

Target: side abs

A | Stand in split stance and hold low cable

B | Twist torso away from machine and draw cable in to your side

C | Flex at the knees to initiate each rep

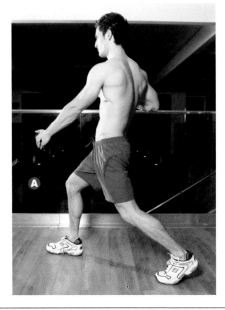

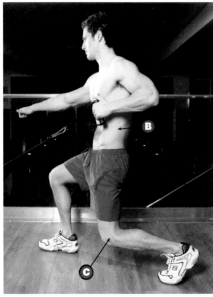

57 One-arm press

Target: side abs

A | Face away from machine and hold high cable in split stance

B | Twist torso and press cable away from your body

C | Flex at the knees to initiate each rep

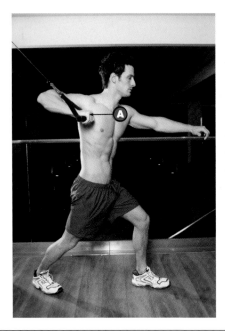

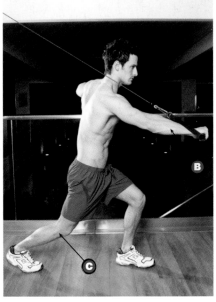

58 **Low cable crunch**

Target: upper abs

A | Lie before a low cable and hold handle in front of face

B | Curl shoulders off floor

C | Pause at top and lower slowly to the start

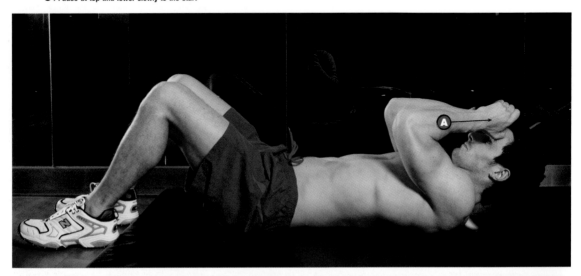

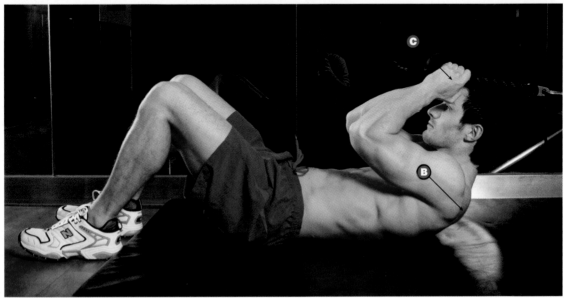

59 ► Cable reverse crunch

Target: lower abs

A | Lie with feet towards low cable and attach cable to ankles

B | Hold thighs vertical and bend knees at 90°

C | Curl your hips off floor and return slowly to the start

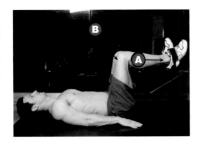

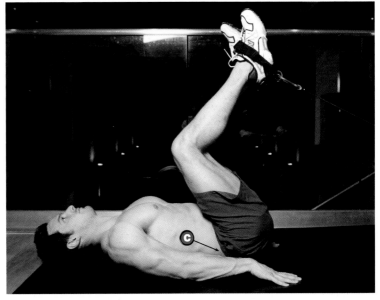

60 ► One-arm high cable crunch

Target: upper abs

A | Kneel before cable and hold handle in one hand in front of face

B | Curl shoulders towards knees without letting body twist to side

C | Pause at bottom, then rise slowly to the start

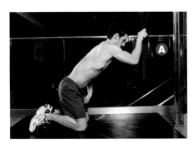

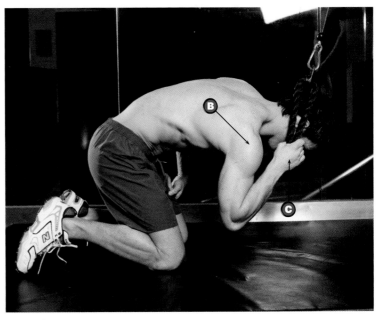

MEDIUM

61 One-arm high cross crunch

Target: side abs

A | Kneel before high cable and hold handle in one hand in front of face

B | Curl shoulders down and twist one elbow towards opposite knee

C | Pause at bottom, then rise slowly to the start

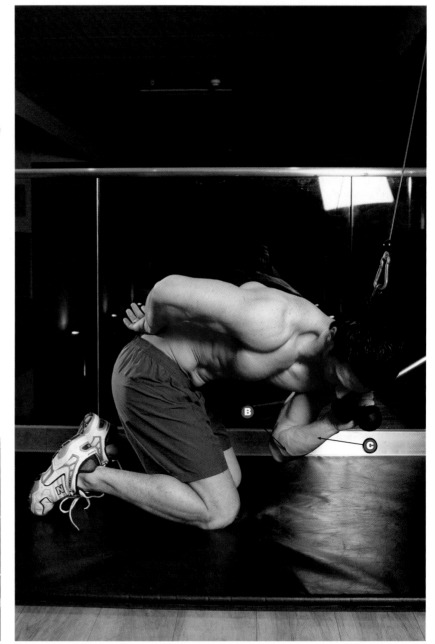

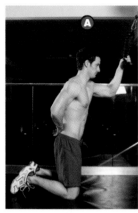

62 Judo throw

Target: upper abs

A | Stand side-on to high cable with wide stance

B | Twist body away from stack and pull cable over shoulder

C | Crunch forward, pulling cable down

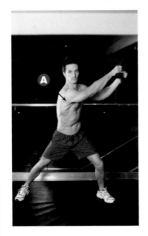 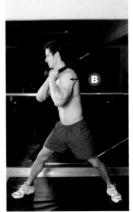

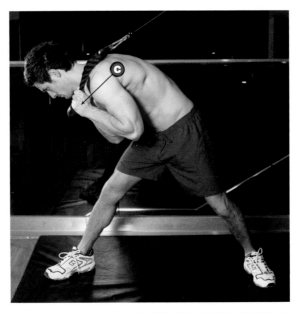

63 Twin cable tuck and crunch

Target: upper and lower abs

A | Lie between twin cables attached to both hands and feet

B | Hold knees and elbows at 90˚

C | Raise shoulders and hips off floor at same time, hold and return

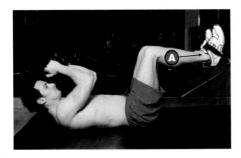

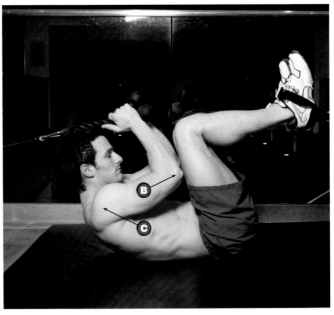

64 Gym ball cable leg raise

Target: lower abs

A I Lie back on a gym ball with cable attached to feet
B I Grab a support for stability and hold legs out in front of you
C I Draw legs up while maintaining stability on ball

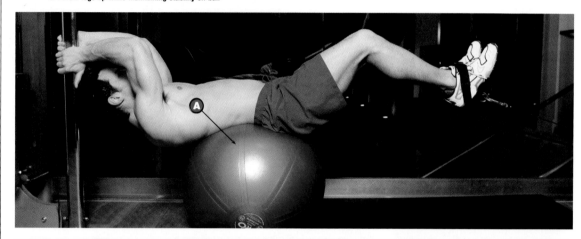

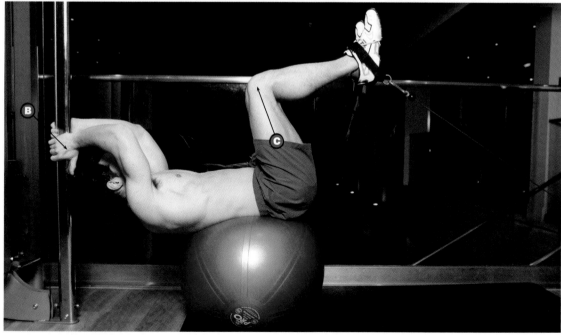

65 High to low cable woodchop

Target: whole core

A | Stand side-on to high cable, then turn torso towards it

B | Draw cable down and across your body, turning torso

C | Keep your back straight and core tensed throughout

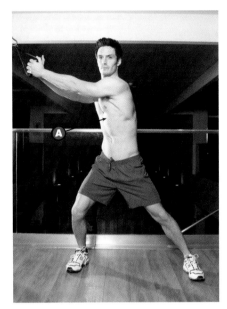
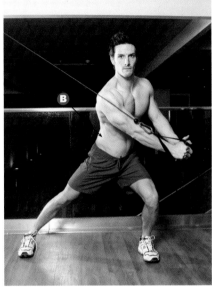

66 Gym ball cable Russian twist

Target: side abs

A | Lie on a gym ball side-on to cable machine

B | Turn torso towards stack, keeping body flat from head to knees

C | With straight arms, draw cable across body to other side

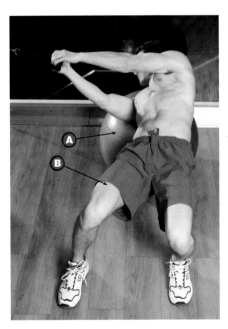
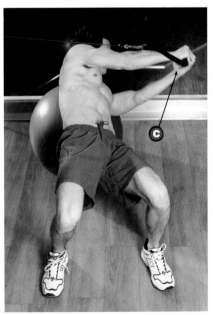

Bar**bell**

More ways to work your abdominals

MEDIUM

67 **Uneven side bends**

Target: side abs

A | Place weight plate on one end of bar only and secure with collar

B | Rest bar across back of shoulders

C | Lean slowly to weighted side and then return to the start

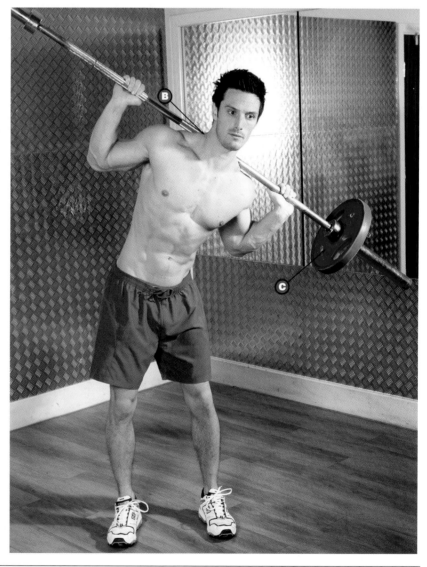

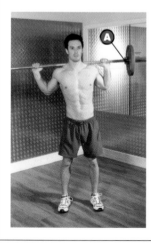

68 ▶ Barbell rollout

Target: lower abs

A | Kneel in front of barbell and grasp it beneath your shoulders

B | Lean forward as far as you can, pushing bar in front of you

C | Return to the start, keeping your back straight throughout

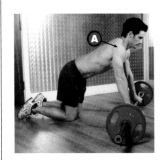
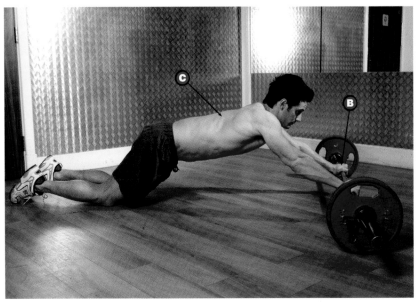

69 ▶ Barbell rotation

Target: whole core

A | Stand with barbell across backs of shoulders

B | Rotate body to one side, keeping your back upright

C | Rotate back and forth, using your abs to control the movement

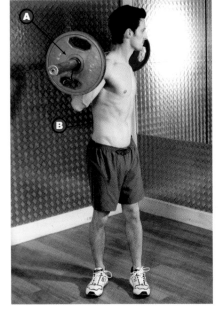
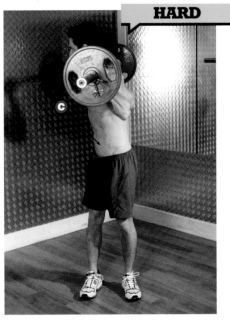

Pull-up/**dip bar**

Lift your bodyweight and hit your abs hard

These three exercises can be performed hanging from a pull-up bar or resting on dip bars

MEDIUM

70 Hanging knee raise

Target: lower abs

A | Hang from pull-up bar or rest on dip bars with feet hanging down

B | Draw knees up to chest

C | Hold for a moment, then lower slowly to the start without swinging

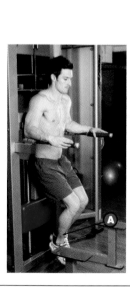

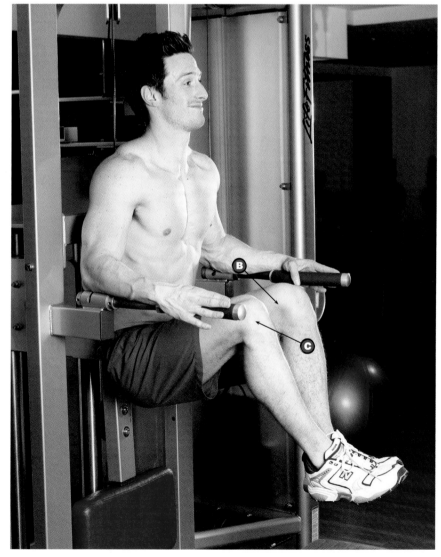

71 Hanging side twist

Target: side abs

A | Hang from pull-up bar or rest on dip bars with feet hanging down

B | Draw knees up and twist to the side

C | Lower slowly to the start and repeat to the other side

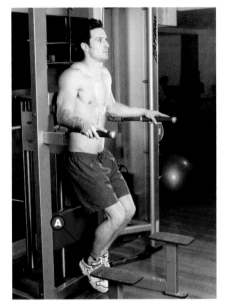
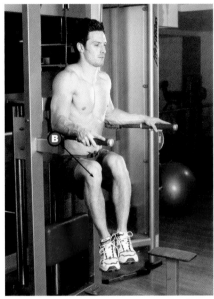

72 Hanging leg raise

Target: lower abs

A | Hang from pull-up bar or rest on dip bars with feet hanging down

B | Keeping your legs straight, raise them out in front of you

C | Pause at the top, then lower slowly to the start

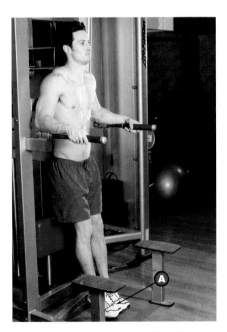

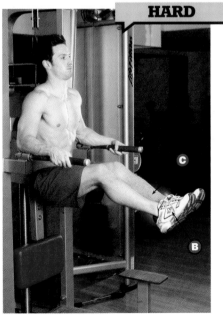

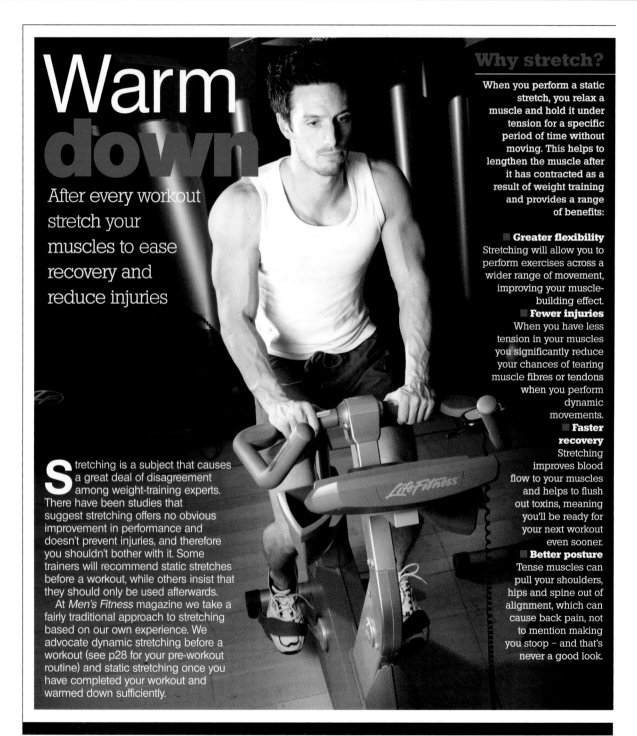

Warm down

After every workout stretch your muscles to ease recovery and reduce injuries

Stretching is a subject that causes a great deal of disagreement among weight-training experts. There have been studies that suggest stretching offers no obvious improvement in performance and doesn't prevent injuries, and therefore you shouldn't bother with it. Some trainers will recommend static stretches before a workout, while others insist that they should only be used afterwards.

At *Men's Fitness* magazine we take a fairly traditional approach to stretching based on our own experience. We advocate dynamic stretching before a workout (see p28 for your pre-workout routine) and static stretching once you have completed your workout and warmed down sufficiently.

Why stretch?

When you perform a static stretch, you relax a muscle and hold it under tension for a specific period of time without moving. This helps to lengthen the muscle after it has contracted as a result of weight training and provides a range of benefits:

■ **Greater flexibility**
Stretching will allow you to perform exercises across a wider range of movement, improving your muscle-building effect.

■ **Fewer injuries**
When you have less tension in your muscles you significantly reduce your chances of tearing muscle fibres or tendons when you perform dynamic movements.

■ **Faster recovery**
Stretching improves blood flow to your muscles and helps to flush out toxins, meaning you'll be ready for your next workout even sooner.

■ **Better posture**
Tense muscles can pull your shoulders, hips and spine out of alignment, which can cause back pain, not to mention making you stoop – and that's never a good look.